Psychiatry on the Stage

How Plays Can Enhance Our Understanding of Psychiatric Conditions

CAROL W. BERMAN

Clinical Assistant Professor of Psychiatry,
NYU Langone Medical Center

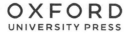

OXFORD
UNIVERSITY PRESS

OXFORD
UNIVERSITY PRESS

Oxford University Press is a department of the University of Oxford. It furthers the University's objective of excellence in research, scholarship, and education by publishing worldwide. Oxford is a registered trade mark of Oxford University Press in the UK and certain other countries.

Published in the United States of America by Oxford University Press
198 Madison Avenue, New York, NY 10016, United States of America.

Library of Congress Cataloging-in-Publication Data
Names: Berman, Carol W., author.
Title: Psychiatry on the stage : how plays can enhance our understanding of
psychiatric conditions / by Carol W. Berman.
Description: New York, NY : Oxford University Press, [2023] |
Includes bibliographical references and index.
Identifiers: LCCN 2022044631 (print) | LCCN 2022044632 (ebook) |
ISBN 9780197622032 (paperback) | ISBN 9780197622056 (epub) |
ISBN 9780197622063 (online)
Subjects: MESH: Medicine in Literature | Psychiatry | Drama | Mental Disorders
Classification: LCC RC489.P7 (print) | LCC RC489.P7 (ebook) | NLM WM 49 |
DDC 616.89/1653—dc23/eng/20221209
LC record available at https://lccn.loc.gov/2022044631
LC ebook record available at https://lccn.loc.gov/2022044632

DOI: 10.1093/med/9780197622032.001.0001

Printed by Marquis Book Printing, Canada

To Barbara and Marty for their loving support

Contents

Foreword

Perry Brass

"We are such stuff/as dreams are made on; and our little life/Is rounded with a sleep," says Prospero in Shakespeare's last play that he wrote alone, *The Tempest*, in one of the most beautiful speeches ever delivered by a human on a stage. When I first heard this great speech, I could not understand why Prospero says that we, meaning humans and actors, are "such stuff as dreams are made on," rather than "of." Aren't we of the evanescence that dreams are made *of*?

Yet Shakespeare as the consummate artist instinctively tells us something deeper, more disquieting—and that is truly what theater is about. In this book about the intersection of psychiatry and theater, Carol Berman explains theater to us in a psychiatric format, showing us how plays from the Greeks and Shakespeare to the nineteenth century and more contemporary drama both presage the theories of psychoanalysis and in many ways embody them.

How theater does this is very simple. The Greeks knew it, and everyone else who has ever "played the boards," as a creator or performer, knows it. It is done by externalizing what is deepest, most hidden, maybe most frightening, and at times even most hilarious. Or, as Berman says: "Basically, Freud wanted to make unconscious thoughts conscious. Plays do the same thing in many ways, projecting our unconscious ideas and wishes onto the stage. Our unconscious desires and needs are expressed by the actors." In good theater, the line between hilarity and horror is thin, just as the line between fear and attraction is.

In theater, instilling fear and attraction at the same time is a constant device—we are all terrified of our own attractions, as well as our own most deep-seated fears, and it is the work of both the playwright and the therapist to work with these twisting strands of emotional DNA that are present in all humans. One of Berman's great steps in this book is that she sees the theater going on within analysis and therapy itself: how the therapist, or analyst, is actually producing theater, the same way that Freud himself "worked the audience" (i.e., the medical world) by tailoring his own theories to please it. Although he believed, just as many playwrights did, that seduction—and sexual abuse—in all its guises and moments was paramount in producing neuroses, he did not want to skew the emerging world of psychoanalysis so strongly in that direction: It would be too frightening and distasteful to the bourgeois Austrian society Freud trained and moved in.

In all instances of theater and analysis, one at a certain point reaches the feeling that both of these pursuits are simply very graspable "handles" necessary for understanding the world—that is, for people in need of healing and understanding, to have a sheltered place to rest and look at themselves. This book does provide a sheltered place—it is as much a layman's guidebook to the many different branches of psychiatry and analysis as it is to the plays that Berman takes apart to show us the psychological underpinnings of them. Thus, we get a capsule view of Freudianism, Jungian analysis, Adlerian thought, Gestalt therapy, Reichian therapy, and beyond to people like Melanie Klein. We also get a glimpse at basic personality disorders, like OCD (obsessive-compulsive disorder), PPD (paranoid personality disorder), and BPD (borderline personality disorder), among others. Berman illustrates these disorders through plays like *Glengarry Glen Ross, Othello, The Glass Menagerie*, and the plays of Lanford Wilson.

What Berman has given us here is an extensive and very worked out view of both world theater and the psychological problems that so many of us have. The book brings a lump to your throat when you read her chapter "Depression and Bipolar Disorder," and she uses the very successful plays of Lanford Wilson, Chekhov, Arthur Miller, and even Christopher Durang to illustrate this potentially even fatal diagnosis of depression. Having gone through the duress of having a depressed husband, sister, and mother, I found her guide through this situation both cogent and useful.

"When a person suffers from depression," Berman says, "his thoughts are narrowed down into a dark tunnel. Depressed people actually have fewer neurotransmitters flowing through their brains, so that their thoughts are scanty and limited. Antidepressants, electroconvulsive therapy (ECT), and other brain stimulation techniques such as ketamine infusions all increase neurotransmission and bring relief to depressed patients."

Sometimes, though, what the depressed person needs is something to get them even temporarily out of the source of depression, to give them the catharsis and lifting of spirits that is necessary. Theater can do that; it can provide the keyhole to another plane of experience, understanding, and the scattered, painful, nuts and bolts of existence. Carol Berman has given us all of these things in this new book with a new twist on psychiatry and analysis. But enough of me; it's time to begin.

Acknowledgments

I would like to thank Barbara Eubanks for her dedication and help in typing up this book and offering many comments and inspiring ideas.

I totally appreciate my Dramatists' Guild Playwright's Group (DGPG), who meet with me every Wednesday. We were meeting in person but now, after the pandemic, we Zoom.

Thanks also go out to NYU Langone Medical Center, where I have the privilege of being a clinical assistant professor in psychiatry. It is there I mentored so many students, residents, and colleagues who encouraged me.

Thanks to the editorial staff at Oxford University Press.

About the Author

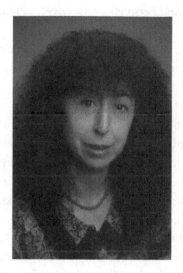

As a preeminent member of the medical community and recently elected Life Distinguished Fellow of the American Psychiatric Association, Dr. Carol W. Berman is that rare and courageous physician who—much like the late prolific and beloved neurologist Dr. Oliver Sachs—is not afraid to draw on her own artistic and intuitive powers to enhance her scientific approach and engage her patients in a deeper level of healing and self-empowerment.

Carol Berman grew up in Los Angeles and studied at the University of California at Berkeley as an undergraduate. Once she moved to New York, she attended New York University (NYU) Medical School. Her residency in psychiatry was spent at St. Luke's–Roosevelt Hospital. In 1986, she returned to NYU to accept a research fellowship at NYU Langone Medical Center, where she remains as a clinical assistant professor in psychiatry. She is also in private practice in New York City. When she is not writing or treating patients, she paints in acrylics, oils, or watercolors.

As an author and playwright, Carol Berman is at home in both nonfiction and fiction. For seven years, she wrote a monthly column on mental health for the *Huffington Post*, and several of her short stories have been published in literary magazines. In addition, she currently serves on the editorial board of *The Bellevue Literary Review*.

Dr. Berman's nonfiction books include *100 Questions and Answers About Panic Disorder*, first published by Jones and Bartlett in 2005 and reissued in its second edition in 2010; and *Personality Disorders*, published by Lippincott, Williams & Wilkins in 2009. Dr. Berman's third book, *Surviving Dementia: A Clinical and Personal Perspective*, came out in 2016, published by Springer Press.

Taming the Negative Introject, her latest book on empowering patients to take control of their mental health, was published in 2019 and is available now from Amazon.com and Taylor & Francis.

One of her theater pieces, *Under the Dragon*, was presented in The Workshop at the Neighborhood Playhouse in New York City. Then, she had a staged reading of the play at the United Nations in 2003, and the JCC (Jewish Community Center) in Manhattan. The film of the play was shown at the American Psychiatric Association Conference in San Francisco in 2019. In this comedy, a woman psychiatrist with bipolar disorder is stalked by her patient, whom she falls in love with and believes he has committed suicide.

Her next play, *Sunshine Sally*, was produced in 2004 at the Workshop at the Neighborhood Playhouse. It's the story of a California hippy transported to New York City who is trying to adapt to her boyfriend's traditional family on Thanksgiving. Her troubles include being a vegetarian and fighting with authority figures. At the end, a turkey flies and a baby is delivered.

Professional Misconduct was produced by Egoactus Company in 2009. In this drama, an emergency room doctor starts hallucinating and is locked up in the psych ward in his own hospital. Consequently, he loses his license and has to appear before the Office of Professional Medical Conduct to try to get it back.

Brownstone Breakdown was produced by Egoactus Company in 2010. This comedy is based on real events about tenants' rights in 1983. Many characters in a small brownstone in midtown Manhattan band together to confront a Mafioso landlord who wants to throw them all out or else!

In the Kingdom of Sam, we enter the world of Sandra, an artist whose husband, Sam, has had a stroke. Sam is so diminished that he imagines himself a king accompanied by a jester, Manny. This story is similar to *King Lear*. Sam has to fight for his survival as King Lear did. This play was presented as part of a Stagecraft Festival, a play festival at the Manhattan Repertory Theater.

Parking Lot 63 had a run at the Hudson Guild Theater during their summer festival in 2015. This is the story of a 13-year-old girl who, although sexually abused herself, is able to rescue another young girl from sexual slavery.

Light My Fire was presented as a staged reading at the Dixon Place Theater in June 2019. Set in the turbulent 1960s in Berkley, California, two college students discover sex, drugs, and rock and roll.

Double Blind ran at Theater Row on 42nd Street in New York City in spring 2022. Diane, a young psychiatry resident at a big city hospital, discovers that her chief, Dr. Render, and Big Pharma are experimenting on mental patients by giving them dangerous medications. She tries to save Emily, a woman with schizophrenia, with the help of her boyfriend, Bert, a lawyer, and Dr. Sanders, the head of the emergency room.

Introduction

The first time I saw a play was when I was twelve and a nerdy math major in junior high. Our class went to downtown Los Angeles and saw a Shakespeare play. I forget which one we saw (I only remember it was about a king), but I fell in love with theater right then and there. They were talking in some weird variation of English to my mind, but the actors were so good I could immediately understand what they meant. I came from a working-class family, and the only thing I'd watched until then was TV or a movie. I probably developed a neural network at that time, which connected the scientific part of my brain to my artistic part.

After that, I convinced my father to take me to another play. We saw *Rain* by John Colton, which was based on a short story by Somerset Maugham, about a missionary who falls in love with a prostitute and winds up raping her. The sexuality was intense and over my prepubescent head, but my father enjoyed it and didn't care if I learned about sex this way.

Then, in the 1970s when I moved back to New York City (where I was born), I could go to the theater whenever I had the time or money. Medical school, psychiatric residency, my fellowship, and my private practice all kept me busy for years. As a result, it wasn't until 2000 that I started writing my own plays. Fortunately, I lived around the corner from the Neighborhood Playhouse, the home of the Meisner technique. Sanford Meisner was a student of the famous Lee Strasberg, but he broke away and established his own method of truth in acting. I took playwriting classes and one acting class there. It was a fantastic education. We used actors from the school to put on our plays.

The Neighborhood Playhouse produced two of my plays, *Under the Dragon* and *Sunshine Sally*. The first was in 2003 and the second in 2004. I also met directors who saw my work and then took me to other venues to produce *Professional Misconduct*, *Brownstone Breakdown*, *Parking Lot 63* and *Light My Fire*. Now, I'm working with an inspiring group of playwrights who call themselves DGPG (Dramatists Guild Playwrights Group). We are currently presenting plays and participating in many festivals.

Once I began writing plays, I could see the psychological underpinnings so clearly. *Oedipus Rex*, one of the Greek classics, is the basis for Freud's Oedipus complex. A boy loves his mother and wants to eliminate his father: how simple a complex, how disturbing, but how true. In the original story, Oedipus, who doesn't realize who his parents are, inadvertently winds up marrying his mother and killing his father. When he gains knowledge of his parentage, he gouges his eyes out in horror. He doesn't want to see anymore. Modern plays that follow this pattern are *Desire Under the Elms*, *Hamlet*, and similar works.

The Electra complex, so named by Jung, falls under the same category as the Oedipus complex, only this time the girl falls for her father and wishes to kill her mother. In psychiatry, we call them both the Oedipus complex. Other plays that illustrate this complex, besides Sophocles' *Electra*, include Eugene O' Neill's *Mourning Becomes Electra*, Sartre's *The Flies*, Alfaro's *Eletricidad*, and Kennedy's *Electra and Orestes*.

In classical Greek drama, according to Aristotle in his *Poetics*, the term *catharsis* refers to the purification and purgation of emotion through art. In psychiatry, catharsis refers to the working out of suppressed or repressed emotions through psychotherapy. In theater, catharsis refers to the effect of tragedy or comedy on the audience. As the audience watches the drama, for example, unrealized emotions in audience members will be projected on the characters in the play. For instance, in *The Glass Menagerie*, through Laura, an introverted and perhaps autistic young woman who prefers to concentrate on her glass figurines and thereby block out the world, audience members may relate to their own introversion and isolation feelings and work them out.

The concept of "transference," in the psychiatric context, refers to a patient transferring feelings onto the therapist so that the therapist may represent the patient's own father, mother, spouse, or siblings. In theater, we project onto the actors our feelings about our family members as well. For example, in William's *The Rose Tattoo*, Serafina becomes our mother as she deals with her rebellious daughter, and we feel the transference of our emotions toward her.

Researchers are demonstrating that neural networks are the future. We already install something similar in supercomputers to compute at top speeds. We humans process the world through our neural networks. We can use these networks for creativity and to bring together what used to be called our right and left brains. The right brain was thought to be associated with art, literature, music, and theater, and the left brain was for math, science, and other analytical subjects. We have discovered it's not so simple since both hemispheres of our brain are operating to process everything together.

Unfortunately, funding for theater and other arts has almost dried up in the United States. The National Endowment for the Arts (NEA) was established in 1965 to make sure all Americans had access to the arts. Our government wanted to eliminate the NEA entirely, but presently its budget is being reviewed. Americans admire inventions of a practical nature. We invented airplanes, computers, phones, and many other things. However, we lag behind other countries in paying respect to the arts. I've been impressed by former Soviet satellite countries, like Romania, that fund the arts so well.

Theater is not a lost art as some claim. Here in New York City, theater is alive and well. During the pandemic it was on pause, but I'm sure theater will have a revival very soon. I believe that theater promotes mental health and stimulates our neural networks. Hence, this book elaborates theater's beneficial effects and psychiatric connections.

1

The Greeks

When I was first in training as a psychiatric resident, my supervisor asked me if I understood the Oedipus complex. We were discussing a patient of mine who completely mystified me with his procrastination. At that point in my life, I had seen few plays, and I had to admit that I hadn't seen Sophocles's play *Oedipus Rex*. My conception of the Oedipus complex was vague. My supervisor, a psychoanalyst of some renown, promised me that if I could grasp this complex, I would understand not only my present patient, but also many others to come.

"Is it that my patient wants to sleep with his mother and kill his father?" I asked, hoping that my simple formulation would at least touch on some of the problems.

"Exactly," said my supervisor and then further elaborated about Oedipus, who was raised by strangers and didn't know who his parents were. He winds up marrying his mother, Jocasta, and slaying his father, Laius. Excited by this explanation, I went home and read Sophocles's play, which I wouldn't be able to see live on stage for many years.

My patient, a graduate student, was stuck writing his PhD thesis as well as in his life. He couldn't date or move on in any way. His mother had been doting and too involved with him, while his father was aggressive and cruel to him. He had dreams of killing an older man, which I interpreted as his desire to rid himself of his father so he could move on with his life. I couldn't come right out and give my patient the simple formulation I'd given my supervisor. He would think I was deranged. Slowly after about one year of psychotherapy, he began to recognize his anger at his father and sexual attraction to his mother. Before he completed his treatment, he finished his thesis and began dating. This was my first success in helping a patient understand himself.

I was amazed that the Greeks figured out this basic human dynamic in 400 BC. Freud analyzed this play and used it as a basis for his concepts. Many Greek artifacts and writings had come to light during the time he was conceptualizing his theories. Archaeological discoveries had captured the imagination of the public in turn-of-the-century Vienna, Austria.

"What about the Electra complex?" I asked my supervisor when I was treating a woman patient who displayed many of the same features as my Oedipus patient.

"You mean the case in which the woman wants to have sex with her father and kill her mother?"

"Yes."

"We call that the Oedipal complex as well."

I didn't protest at the time since I knew Freud was paternalistic, and the Viennese society he lived in, the late 1800s and early 1900s, was doubly so. I also was aware that my supervisor was a male chauvinist, and I didn't want to antagonize him. Currently many psychiatrists disregard Freud's concepts because of his failure to view women realistically and sympathetically. Jung, on the other hand, wanted to keep the term "the Electra complex" to explain a woman's attraction to her father and rejection of her mother, but Freud overruled him at the time.

Psychoanalysts consider the positive Oedipal complex the case in which the child is attracted to the opposite sex parent, while the negative Oedipal complex is when the child desires the same sex parent. Freud believed that the child's identification with the same sex parent is the successful outcome of the complex, and the unsuccessful identification results in homosexuality. Now, we don't think homosexuality stems from unsuccessful identification with the same sex parent. Many studies have attempted to explain homo-sexuality. Theories have ranged from considering various brain structures to be different in homosexuals to hormonal variations, to genes, or to environ-mental causes. We're still not sure what makes individuals choose homosex-uality, but it's considered a variation on the normal.

Greek drama originated with people celebrating Dionysus, the god of wine and fertility. The Greeks had boisterous festivals when the seasons changed. The people sang, danced, prayed, drank, joked, had sex, and gave thanks to their gods. The Greeks reveled in the lovely spring and summer months. Then they were sad when winter came and their crops died. Comedies stemmed from *komos*, which means revel, so these probably originated in the spring and summer. Comedies were produced at that time of the year and then the tragedies when winter came.

It was in the golden age of Greece that Aeschylus and his successors, Euripides and Sophocles, produced their tragedies. Aeschylus was the first of Athens' three great playwrights. Aeschylus produced his first play in 499 BC. Like all the Greeks, he had an amazing ability to understand psychological interactions. He was born to an aristocratic family. Many of his plays deal with theology and important questions like the meaning of justice.

In *Agamemnon*, Clytemnestra is the protagonist who carries out a murderous revenge on her husband, Agamemnon, for violating their home. Agamemnon had to kill their daughter, Iphigenia, as a sacrifice to the goddess Artemis so that his fleet could pass for the Trojan War. This king returns from war after ten years. He has Cassandra, his trophy, in his chariot. She famously predicts many things when she goes into a trance, including her own death and the king's death. Apollo put a curse on Cassandra, so that she could predict the future but no one will believe her. Clytemnestra does kill the king, and with her lover, Aegisthus, explains that this is a twofold revenge because Agamemnon's father, Atreus, killed and cooked Aegisthus's brothers and fed them to their father. Revenge and murder are prominent in many Greek plays. In ordinary conscious life, we usually don't achieve revenge or murder our enemies, but in Greek tragedies our unconscious negative feelings are fully expressed. Even though the first few moments may feel rewarding to the person, psychologically we have found that instead of extinguishing hostility, revenge actually prolongs the unpleasantness of the original offense. Instead of delivering justice, revenge often creates only a cycle of retaliation. Agamemnon acts on hereditary guilt and the curses on his family brought on by crimes against them. So, Aeschylus wrote two more plays in this cycle of revenge that trapped his characters.

Eating the enemy or other people happens often in Greek stories. Freud would refer to this cannibalism as regressing to the oral–sensory stage, which occurs in the first year of an infant's life. This stage concerns trust versus distrust. Certainly Atreus did not trust Aegisthus's brothers and feeding them to their father was the ultimate insult to their father.

The Choephore, Aeschylus's second play in this trilogy, takes place ten years later. Prince Orestes, Agamemnon's son, and his friend Pylades are at the prince's father's tomb when he sees his sister, Electra, still mourning for their father. He vows to take vengeance on his father's murderers. Electra and Orestes team up. They realize that their mother, Clytemnestra, has sent libations for the king's tomb because in her guilt about killing the king she has nightmares. In one nightmare, Clytemnestra gives birth to a serpent, which she suckles. Orestes recognizes himself in this dream as the serpent.

Jung would have agreed with Orestes about the symbolism and added that the serpent is a male symbol of fertility. Orestes and Pylades plan to sneak into the palace and kill his mother and her lover, Aegisthus. Orestes puts on a disguise before he visits his mother to tell her that he, Orestes, is dead. She seems to mourn, but the chorus reveals that his mother is lying. She is not that disturbed by her son's death. However, Cilissa, who was Orestes's old nurse, overhears this news. She is truly in mourning for her beloved Orestes. Cilissa runs to Aegisthus urging him to hurry out and meet the witness to Orestes's death. Orestes and Pylades kill Aegisthus and then Clytemnestra, even after she pleads for her life. Orestes understands that his matricide will haunt him. He vows to remain childless and wifeless rather than have such a wife as his mother was.

The chorus serves many purposes in Greek plays. First, the chorus comments on actions and events and supplies additional information that the audience needs to fully understand the play. Second, they are the collective conscious and unconscious of the characters. We can't read Orestes's mind, but the chorus supplies us with his fears and plans. They tell us the truth about Clytemnestra's feelings. They also spur on the characters to their deeds.

The Eumenides was the third tragedy in Aeschylus's trilogy. Pythia, the high priestess of the temple of Apollo at Delphi, enters the temple at first but then dashes out because she's had a terrible vision of Orestes surrounded by the Furies. Then Orestes, Apollo, Hermes, and the half-asleep Furies exit the temple. Apollo pledges to help Orestes and sends Hermes with him to Athena's citadel. Meanwhile Clytemnestra's ghost stirs up the Furies to get her son. The Furies fight with Apollo and blame him for causing Orestes to commit matricide. Apollo retorts that revenge had to be taken for Agamemnon's death. They all set out to visit Athena, who is at the Acropolis in Athens. When they arrive, Athena wants to hear both sides of the story. When she hears Orestes and then the Furies, she looks for a jury since the case is so complicated she can't decide by herself who's right. Twelve citizens return with Athena. Apollo testifies in front of this court. The chorus presents the facts of the case. At the end, Athena rules in favor of Orestes, and the Furies spew their anger at the goddess. She promises them their own place underground. They become the Eumenides (the kind ones) and bless Athens. It is as if the negative introject, represented by the Furies, is subdued and becomes benign. It's a quick turnaround for the Furies. They go from furious to restrained in a matter of moments.

Euripides was an antisocial loner born around 484 BC. Even after he was a famous playwright, he chose to live in a cave rather than in the city. His father consulted an oracle when he was born; the oracle predicted "crowns of victory" for his son. Euripides studied athletics, painting, and philosophy before writing plays. Euripides was married and had three sons, although he was accused of misogyny. It's ironic because he wrote sensitive studies of women, like Medea and Electra.

Electra was written by Euripides in about 413 BC. It continues the story of Agamemnon's (the king's) children, Iphigenia, Orestes, Chrysothemis, and, of course, Electra. The whole family has a curse on it, stemming from Electra's great-grandfather, Atreus, who angered the gods. When the king returns from the battle in Troy, he is murdered by his wife's (Clytemnestra's) lover, Aegisthus, who had also planned to murder Electra since she was an obstacle to his ambitions. Electra is saved by her mother. Then she is married off to a peasant so her children will not be noble and have the ability to rise to the throne. Her brother, Orestes, appears in disguise until an old servant recognizes him, and then the brother and sister reunite. Electra promises to kill her mother, while Orestes kills Aegisthus. In the end, Electra manages to kill her mother with the help of her brother. Thus, we have the Electra complex, or the woman's Oedipus complex.

Another powerful story of family dynamics by Euripides is *Medea*. It opens as a romance between Jason and Medea. Medea has helped Jason acquire the Golden Fleece, a symbol of authority and kingship, to help place him on the throne in Thessaly. However, even after all she has done, the Argonaut Jason jilts Medea, forsakes their two sons, and marries King Creon's daughter. Medea, her nurse, and the chorus all complain about the injustice that women face. Creon exiles Medea and her children because he fears her magical powers. Medea plots revenge. When Jason mocks her anger, Medea puts a curse on him and Creon. She then conspires with Aegeus, the king of Athens, and promises to kill Creon's daughter as well as her own children.

To interpret Medea psychologically, I want to consider object relations theory, which simply is a theory that shows us how relationships with others, especially the mother, determine our personality. The theory includes real and external people, as well as internal "objects." Adults relate to others based on their experiences as an infant. Images of people and events turn into "objects" in the unconscious that the self carries. Then the self uses these objects to predict people's behavior.

The first such object is the mother or primary caregiver. Fairbairn[1] challenged Freud's drive theory with object relations. He assumed that our unconscious develops as a child and incorporates disassociated memories of abuse and neglect that are impossible to tolerate consciously. Attachment to an abusive caregiver is then possible and necessary since children are so dependent. They have no choice but to attach to such parents. In his three-part model, there is the central conscious ego and two unconscious parts: an antilibidinal ego (rejecting parts of the "object") and a libidinal ego (relating to the exciting, loving part). The last two remain in the unconscious but can emerge to take over the person's central ego. When they emerge, the other person is seen as loving or rejecting—thus exhibiting transference. Fairbairn said this is how the defense mechanism of splitting occurs, especially in borderline personality disorder.

Medea becomes the antilibidinal ego when she destroys her own children. She is acting out of revenge against her husband, Jason, who has rejected her in order to marry the king's daughter. Usually, mothers act with the libidinal ego, the loving part of themselves. How shocking for anyone to view Medea's actions in Euripides's eponymous play. We might unconsciously hold these views in our minds, but very few people act on them. How amazing it is that the ancient Greeks not only conceived of these possibilities but also acted them out on stage.

In 408 BC, Euripides wrote *The Orestes*, another story about Agamemnon's family. At the beginning, Electra justifies the killing of their mother and her lover by her brother, Orestes. She grieves for her brother, Orestes, who is prostrate with mental torment. The gods have given him "madness." He can't eat or wash. He just stays in his filthy cloak, raving and lost in "limbo." The people of Argos, the city they are in, will either stone them or cut their heads off. Electra wants Menelaus's (her uncle's) fleet to arrive from Troy. Helen, Electra and Orestes's aunt, half-heartedly comforts her niece and nephew. Helen tells Electra to make a sacrificial offering (of hair and wine) for her mother, Clytemnestra. Electra wants Helen's daughter, Hermione, to do it. Orestes wakes up after a long sleep and seems to be coherent, but soon the Furies grab him and once again he is raving. Menelaus arrives in town, but he grieves Clytemnestra's and Agamemnon's deaths. He wants to greet his nephew, Orestes, who explains that his conscience threw away his reason. Orestes has terrible guilt, and when his grandfather spits at him,

[1] Fairbairn, W. R. D., *Psychoanalytical Studies of the Personality* (London: Routledge, 1952).

he feels worse. But then Orestes turns the tables and blames the old man for siring such evil children. The grandfather stirs the crowds to stone his grandchildren. The mob goes back and forth in their feelings toward the doomed brother and sister. Finally, Apollo, the god of healing, oracles, and sunlight, intervenes. He orders Orestes to be tried for matricide and then to marry his cousin, Hermione, and rule Argos. Pylades will wed Electra. Apollo takes the blame for Orestes's crime. Helen becomes a goddess and is taken to the throne of Zeus. *Deus ex machina* applies often in Greek plays. It means "God out of the machine" and is a plot device whereby a seemingly insolvable problem is resolved by an unlikely occurrence, such as the gods intervening in human affairs. In the Greek times, they actually employed a machine to drop a deity onto the stage to help resolve problems in the story. The machine was a type of crank, and it represented heaven, the divine abode of the gods.

I find it interesting that Orestes is "mad" with guilt and "mad" because the Furies cause it. Of course, in 400 BC, Euripides had no idea what causes "madness" or the loss of reason. To blame it on outside forces under these circumstances makes perfect sense.

The Trojan Women (415 BC) by Euripides is narrated from a female point of view. Each woman from the Trojan royal house comes forward to tell her tale of suffering at the hands of the invaders. It is the day after the Greeks have taken Troy.

The women are just property to be claimed by victorious Greeks. Hecuba, the queen, goes to Odysseus; Andromache, Hector's widow and Hecuba's daughter-in-law, to Pyrrhus (Achilles' son). Cassandra (the prophetess who is never believed) goes to Agamemnon (the general). There is no plot, but a lot of misery is voiced by the women. Helen is to be taken back to Greece and killed there, but she seduces her husband, Menelaus, to spare her life. Children are sacrificed. Unfortunately, after wars the male conquerors do treat women like this. However, *The Trojan Women* also shows male fantasies of having power over women and using them like property. Biologically, this makes perfect sense: Males need to inseminate females to continue the human race. If males have control of females, they can accomplish this without all the niceties of civilization and societal rules. Throughout history, females have been subjugated in this manner, and even to this day, there are many societies in which women are treated as second-class citizens.

Euripides saw this firsthand since Athens and Sparta fought for control of Greece and perpetuated so much war in his time. Supposedly, he had two terrible marriages in which both his wives were unfaithful. Yet in *The Trojan*

Women, he is clearly on the side of the women as he portrays their agonies. Even so, he ended up alone in a cave writing plays.

Sophocles, the third great tragedian of Athens, was probably born in 496 BC. By the age of 28, he won contests over Euripides and Aeschylus. His themes of sadness, folly, and regret registered with Athenians and then the world. He wrote the incredible stories of *Oedipus Rex*, *Oedipus at Colonus*, and *Antigone*.

In *Antigone*, Eteocles and Polyneices, Oedipus's sons, kill each other fighting for the throne of Thebes. Oedipus's brother-in-law, Creon, takes the throne when they die. Creon declares that Eteocles will be buried but not Polyneices. The latter will be left outside to be picked apart by animals. Antigone and Ismene, sisters to Oedipus's sons, discuss what to do with Polyneices's body. Antigone wants to bury it, but Ismene says not to go against Creon. Antigone states that if it's a choice between human law and sacred law, she'll go with the sacred. She's brought before Creon, who accuses her and her sister of disobeying him. Antigone pleads her sister's case, and then her bridegroom-to-be, Creon's son Haemon, pleads for her. Creon spares Ismene but throws Antigone into a cave to die. Tiresias, a blind prophet, begs Creon to bury Polyneices and to free Antigone. The tragedy ends with Haemon killing himself, Antigone hanging herself, and Eurydice, Creon's wife, killing herself.

In the *Frogs* (405 BC), Aristophanes has the god Dionysus going down to Hades (the underworld) to find a good poet to bring back to Athens. There's a debate between the dead playwrights Euripides and Aeschylus. Dionysus brings back Aeschylus since he's wiser and Euripides is only clever. Dionysus has a slave, Xanthias, who is smarter than him. The frogs are the chorus, and they annoy Dionysus, who debates them.

Dionysus (Bacchus for the Romans) is the Greek god of winemaking, of fertility, and of religious ecstasy and theater.

Aristophanes also wrote *Lysistrata* (411 BC), a comedy expressing women's role in society. Women in general are represented by Calonice, who is an earthy hedonist. Lysistrata, however, is an extraordinary woman with an evolved sense of individual and social responsibility. She has convened an antiwar meeting of women from various Greek city states that are at war with each other. She confides in her friend, Calonice, her concerns for the female sex. The women arrive.

Lysistrata persuades (with Lampito's help) the women to withhold sex from their men as a means of forcing them to conclude the Peloponnesian war. The women are reluctant, but finally convinced, they seal their vows with a solemn oath around a wine bowl. Lysistrata chooses the words, and Calonice repeats them on behalf of the other women. It is a long and detailed oath in which the women abjure all their sexual pleasure.

The old women of Athens seize control of the Acropolis at Lysistrata's instigation since it holds the state treasury, without which the men cannot fund their war. Lampito goes off to spread the word, and the other women lock themselves in the Acropolis to await the men's response.

A Chorus of Old Men arrives, intent on burning down the gate of the Acropolis if the women do not open up. Encumbered with heavy timbers, inhaling smoke, and burdened with old age, they prepare to assault the gate when a Chorus of Old Women arrives, bearing pitchers of water. The Old Women complain about the difficulty getting the water, but they are ready to defend the younger women. Threats are exchanged, water beats fire, and the Old Men are soaked.

The magistrate then arrives with the police. He expounds on the hysterical nature of women, their love of wine, promiscuous sex, and exotic cults, but most of all he blames men for poor supervision of their women. He has come for silver from the state treasury to buy oars for the fleet, and he instructs his Scythians to begin opening the gate. However, they are quickly overwhelmed by groups of unruly women.

Lysistrata restores order, and she allows the magistrate to question her. She explains the frustrations that women feel at a time of war when the men make stupid decisions that affect everyone, and she further complains that their wives' opinions are not listened to. She drapes her headdress over him, gives him a basket of wool, and tells him that war will be a woman's business from now on. She then explains the pity she feels for young, childless women, aging at home while the men are away on endless campaigns. When the magistrate points out that men also age, she reminds him that men can marry at any age, whereas a woman has only a short time before she is considered too old. She then dresses the magistrate like a corpse for laying out and advises him that he's dead. Outraged at these indignities, he storms off to report the incident to his colleagues, while Lysistrata returns to the Acropolis.

The debate between the Chorus of Old Men and the Chorus of Old Women continues until Lysistrata returns, saying her comrades are deserting the cause on the silliest pretexts. After rallying her comrades and restoring their discipline, Lysistrata again returns to the Acropolis to continue waiting for the men's surrender.

Cinesias, the husband of Myrrhine, arrives, desperate for sex. Lysistrata instructs Myrrhine to torture him. Myrrhine tells Cinesias that she will have sex with him but only if he promises to end the war. He promptly agrees, but Myrrhine gets a bed, then a mattress, then a pillow, then a blanket, then a flask of oil, frustrating her husband with delays. Finally, she disappoints him completely by locking herself in the Acropolis again. The Chorus of Old Men commiserates with the young man with a sad song.

A Spartan herald then appears with an erection scarcely hidden inside his tunic, and he requests to see the ruling council to arrange peace talks. The magistrate, also with an erection, laughs at the herald but agrees that peace talks should begin.

They go off to find the delegates. While they are gone, the Old Women make overtures to the Old Men. The Old Men are content to be comforted and fussed over by the Old Women. The two choruses merge, singing and dancing in unison. Peace talks commence, and Lysistrata introduces the Spartan and Athenian delegates to a gorgeous young woman called Reconciliation. The delegates cannot take their eyes off her, while Lysistrata scolds everyone. The delegates fight over the peace terms, but with Reconciliation before them and the burden of sexual deprivation still heavy on them, they quickly overcome their differences and retire to the Acropolis for celebrations. The war is ended.

Another choral song follows. After a bit of humorous dialogue between tipsy dinner guests, the celebrants all return to the stage for a final round of songs, the men and women dancing together. All sing a merry song in praise of Athene, goddess of wisdom and chastity, whose citadel provided a refuge for the women during the events of the comedy, and whose implied blessing has brought about a happy ending to the play.

Freud would have been delighted with this play that embodied many of his theories. Sexual suppression causing major eruptions in society is just what he would have predicted if women refused to have sex.

What can we conclude from all this patricide, matricide, sibling murder, and violence in general? The Greeks were probably no more aggressive and hostile than any other group of humans. Yet, they wrote about more murders in their dramas than other playwrights, except perhaps Shakespeare. I believe they were mining their unconscious more than other groups. Freud believed the unconscious was a storage space for our suppressed aggressive and sexual drives. The Greeks had only the most primitive science to explain their world, so they turned to philosophy and various gods to explain things.

After living with parents who abuse or punish us excessively, we may want to kill them, but, of course, most of us suppress these desires. Even if parents are loving and caring, they are bound to anger or annoy us, and our primitive child selves want to destroy them. Ancient Greek tragedies acted out these murders for the people. They couldn't kill their parents or siblings or kings or queens so easily, but they could watch this on stage. Another purpose of theater was to teach the audience correct behavior. They learned not to kill because of the dire consequences that resulted: curses on your family, bad fortune for individuals, and the wrath of various gods. Also, killing was always done off stage because it was seen as inappropriate for death to be shown directly within a scene, even if it made the show better.

2

Shakespeare

The mysteries surrounding William Shakespeare (1564–1616) remain with us to this day. How can we account for such profundity from a playwright whose father was an illiterate glover and who only received a grammar school education? And how did he know so much about kings, queens, and royalty? In the heady world of his plays, we witness love, battles, suicide, and revenge, to mention just a few. His knowledge of psychology and his use of it in portraying characters is unbelievably accurate. Was it just an innate ability and wisdom? We'll probably never know.

Let us analyze some of his popular and famous plays.

The Tragedy of Richard III portrays an ugly, deformed man whose physical state matches his mental one. Did his physical disfigurement cause him to have an antisocial personality disorder? He manipulates ruthlessly, murders Henry VI and his son Edward, and then he courts the widow, Lady Anne. He pits his brothers against each other, imprisons his nephews, and generally acts aggressively and outrageously toward everyone. He is unable to feel grief or guilt, true signs of sociopathy. In the last act of the play, Henry Tudor arrives with his army. Before the big battle, all the ghosts of the people Richard murdered appear and prophesy his defeat. This is the only way that his guilt can manifest. Shakespeare did not use a chorus in his plays, but ghosts will do in this case. However, Richard ignores the ghosts and is killed by Henry, who becomes King Henry VII.

The Comedy of Errors is a farce that contains many instances of doubling. There are twin brothers with the same name who have twin servants. Besides providing much amusement and cases of mistaken identity, the doubling allows for splitting, a defense mechanism we see often in psychiatry, in which there is a failure in someone's thinking to bring together the dichotomy of both positive and negative aspects of the self. Instead, the positive self is split off from the negative. In the play, one twin is seen as all good at times and the other as all bad. The narrator of the play, Aegeon, a Syracusan merchant, was shipwrecked with his wife, Aemilia, and their twin babies and twin slaves. Everyone arrives in Ephesus on the same day when they are adults.

Confusion reigns and everyone thinks the sons are crazy as they deal with the doubling. Finally, they all figure it out and rejoice. Imagine the joy of reuniting with a loved one you thought was dead. Doubling is used again in *A Midsummer Night's Dream, Hamlet, King Lear, Twelfth Night or What You Will*. Anne Hathaway, Shakespeare's wife, gave birth to twins shortly after they were married. Perhaps that was his inspiration? Twinning and doubling are popular devices used in plays and currently in movies to show two sides. Or perhaps Shakespeare had trouble synthesizing his positive and negative sides?

Romeo and Juliet shows us how young lovers are caught up in the battles and prejudices of families and society at large. The Montagues and Capulets have been enemies for centuries, unable to resolve their differences. Romeo, a Montague, falls in love with Juliet, a Capulet. They are secretly married by her priest. Many complications ensue, and both lovers eventually kill themselves. Suicide of young people struggling to adapt to their worlds is unfortunately common. Many young people are overwhelmed by life and problems that may seem ordinary to more mature adults, but teens and people in their twenties have never encountered these misfortunes before. Suicidal people talk about suicide and are preoccupied with death. They may stock up on pills, guns, or ropes. Then they withdraw and want to be alone. They can behave in risky ways and say goodbye to loved ones.

The Tragedy of Hamlet, Prince of Denmark, is a type of Oedipus story also. Queen Gertrude, King Hamlet's wife, has hastily married her husband's brother, Claudius, after her king's death. Their son, Prince Hamlet, learns from his father's ghost that Claudius murdered his father. The prince then acts erratically to pretend he's crazy so that he can eventually take revenge on his uncle. Before he does so, he kills Polonius, a father figure. Hamlet watches a play within the play in which he sees a king being killed by poison in his ear, the same way his father was killed. There is so much murdering of fathers in this play that it invokes the Oedipus complex many times. Hamlet has to act crazy to distract everyone from his motives. In the same way a boy would be considered insane if he plans to kill his father or a father figure, this is the classical Oedipal complex.

Othello is a magnificent play revealing how paranoia and jealousy poison every aspect of a life. In psychiatry, we even have the Othello syndrome, a mental condition in which someone is pathologically jealous, falsely believing that their wife/husband or lover is unfaithful. The delusional patient is preoccupied and jealous without proof of the loved one straying. It's a delusional disorder in which the affected person has minimal or insignificant evidence to substantiate claims of infidelity. The Othello syndrome may lead to stalking or violence. In the play *Othello*, the main character is an African prince who loves and secretly marries Desdemona, daughter of a Venetian senator. Iago is a jealous ensign of his general Othello. He's angry that Othello promoted Cassio to lieutenant instead of him, so he tells Desdemona's father, Brabanzino, that Othello and Desdemona eloped. Iago makes trouble throughout the play. Not surprisingly, Othello finally kills Desdemona in a fit of jealousy.

All's Well That Ends Well is a lesser-known Shakespearean play. There are gender role reversals and cynical realism, along with fantasies and delusions. Helena, a low-born ward of a countess, loves Bertram, the countess's son. Helena is able to cure the king of his illness because her father was a doctor, and he taught her some medicine. The king then says he will allow her to marry Bertram, but Bertram doesn't want her. He says he will marry her only if she carries his child and wears his family ring. Then Bertram makes it impossible (or so he thinks) to fulfill his two criteria by leaving for war in Italy before Helena has a chance to sleep with him. Bertram's idea of fun is seducing virgins in Italy. He loves virginal Diana, who doesn't care for him. Diana conceives of a plot to put Helena in bed for sex with Bertram instead of herself. This allows Helena to consummate their marriage and get his ring without Bertram knowing. When Bertram returns home, he wants to marry someone else, but Diana stops him, and Helena (whom he thought was dead) appears. Bertram relents since Helena went to so much trouble to get him——hence, the title of the play, *All's Well That Ends Well*. We can see Bertram as a narcissistic young man, only interested in his own pleasure. Helena perseveres and gets her man, which will elevate her status. However, she goes after an unrequited love, which can be considered a delusion or even obsessive compulsiveness.

Titus Andronicus is a revenge fantasy play. Titus, a general in the Roman Army, presents Tamora, queen of the Goths, as a slave to the new Roman emperor, Saturninus, who takes her as a wife. Tamora vows revenge against Titus for killing her son, Alarbus. He is avenging the deaths of his own sons. Tamora and her two remaining sons vow to get revenge on Titus. Titus wants to marry Lavinia, but she is promised to Bassianus (Saturninus's brother), who gets killed. Lavinia is raped, and her tongue and hands are cut off. She writes the names of her attackers using a stick in her mouth. This horrible act is a type of castration feared by most men and unconsciously thought to be what happened to women by some "stubborn" Freudians. Revenge is a primitive response and defense against aggression. *Titus* is one of Shakespeare's earlier plays.

Gary: A Sequel to Titus Andronicus is an absurd comic play by Taylor Mac that I saw in 2019 on Broadway. It takes place in the aftermath of *Titus Andronicus*. In *Gary*, the bodies were piled high on stage, and servants had to clean up the mess while complaining about Titus and the others.

Measure for Measure is a complex play of morality. The Duke of Vienna, Vincentio, leaves after he appoints his substitute, Angelo. Angelo has an ascetic public image, but he is actually corrupt. He tries to use his new position to get sexual favors from Isabella, a novice nun. Angelo reinstates an old law that states that fornication outside marriage is punishable by death. Juliet has become pregnant by her lover, Claudio. He is thrown into jail to be executed. The lovers had planned to marry, but hadn't gotten past the legal problems. When Isabella goes to intercede for Claudio, her brother, Angelo says he will pardon him if Isabella sleeps with him. She refuses and threatens to tell the world of his corruption, but he says no one will believe her. She schemes with the duke, who is disguised as a friar (he never left town but is sneaking around to see how Angelo handles things), to have Mariana, an old fiancée of Angelo, substitute for her in bed. There is much confusion, in which Isabella thinks her brother has been beheaded, but in the end, justice prevails, all identities are revealed, and Angelo is exposed for the liar he is.

In the play *King Lear*, when King Lear wants to retire, he says he will give whoever loves him the most the biggest share of his realm. He's addressing his three daughters. The oldest, Goneril, declares her love immediately and flatters Lear. Then Regan does the same. Finally Cordelia, the youngest, and his favorite, says she loves Lear so much no words can express it properly. Lear is enraged with this reply, so he disinherits Cordelia and divides his kingdom between Goneril and Regan, which in effect gives their shares to their husbands. Then Lear gets angry at the earl of Kent, who protests the arrangements. The Earl of Kent gets banished. Then of Cordelia's two suitors, the duke of Burgundy and the king of France, the first drops out, and the latter marries her. Lear wants to live with one daughter, Goneril, and then the other, Regan. Both sisters were lying when they said they loved their father, Lear, so much. Goneril disrespects her father when he's with her, so he goes to live with Regan. The Fool (an important character like a jester) tells him the truth, that both sisters are evil. Meanwhile, many machinations of the dukes and earls happen. It turns out that the Fool was right, and Regan also treats

Lear badly. Lear rushes out in a storm and rants. Only the Fool and Kent are still with him. Edgar, a legitimate son of Gloucester, pretends he's a madman, Tom O'Bedlam, and babbles to Lear. Gloucester gets his eyes gouged out by Regan and her husband because he was planning to help reinstate Lear. On the heath, Edgar meets his blinded father, who wants to kill himself. Lear is going crazy or he's senile. Gloucester's illegitimate son, Edmund, is plotting against everyone. Gloucester dies. Goneril commits suicide. Cordelia is killed. Lear dies.

Lear can be seen as a demented man from the beginning of the play. His need for his daughters to declare their love for him causes all the trouble that ensues. He has regressed to the point in which he can't recognize the truth of what his daughters are saying. Cordelia, the one honest one, is ironically discounted. Everyone is deceiving everyone else and struggling for the throne. When Gloucester gets his eyes gouged out, it is similar to Oedipus doing this to himself when he learns the truth about his parents. Freud believed Lear was rejecting death when he rejected Cordelia. At the end, when Lear carries the dead body of Cordelia, he is accepting his own death.[1] Lear can also be seen as a narcissistic personality who always needs people to love and admire him. He doesn't consider anyone else as he rambles around in this play. He expects to be taken care of like a baby by his daughters, but like most children of narcissists, they don't have the capacity to do so. In *King Lear*, they do the opposite of what he wants.

In *Love's Labour's Lost*, King Ferdinand of Navarre turns his court into an academy in order to become famous and defeat Time. He tells three of his lords, Berowne, Dumaine, and Longaville, to swear off the company of women for three years so they can focus on fasting and study. No woman can come within a mile of the court by the king's decree. When the Princess of France arrives with her ladies she can't speak to the king. The king falls in love with the princess anyway and the lords with her ladies. They all watch each other. Finally, Berowne confesses to breaking the oath, saying the only study worthy of mankind is that of love. He and the other men give up their vows. There are disguises, tricks, and ruses, but finally all identities are revealed. The play is about masculine sexual desire and how it is redirected into the need for fame and honor. Women are considered dangerous and to be avoided, even though they are the true objects of men's desires.

---

[1] Freud, Sigmund, *Writings on Art and Literature*, Meridian Crossing Aesthetics (Stanford, CA: Stanford University Press, 1997).

Macbeth is one of the simplest of Shakespeare's play: no subplots and no character so developed that it takes our attention away from Lady Macbeth and Macbeth himself. Macbeth and Banquo are generals of Duncan, the king of Scotland. They meet the three witches on the heath, who tell Macbeth that he will be "thane of Cawdor" (something like an earl) and king after that. Macbeth is so consumed with ambition and spurred on by his wife, that he kills the king and takes the Scottish throne himself. Forced to commit more and more murders to keep his position on top, he becomes a tyrant. A civil war breaks out that kills Macbeth and his lady.

Lady Macbeth famously says: "Out, out, damn spot" and tries to wash her hands clean of Duncan's blood since her husband was so traumatized that he couldn't do it. She then walks and talks in her sleep about the assassination of Duncan. Both Macbeths have disturbed sleep after these murders. The guilt and blood stay with them. Scholars have counted the many, many times Shakespeare mentions blood in this play. When Macbeth returns to the three witches to find out more information, they summon apparitions that recite prophecies. They tell him to beware of Macduff. A bloody child reveals that no one born of woman will be able to harm him, so he feels confident he can't be harmed. What the witches mean is that no one born naturally from a woman can harm him, but Macduff was born in a cesarean section, so he is finally able to kill Macbeth.

While trying to distill Shakespeare's complicated plays into simple plots so I could easily analyze them, I became frustrated. There were so many twists and turns in even such supposedly straightforward stories as *Hamlet* or *Romeo and Juliet* that I was totally surprised. I'd seen so many of the bard's plays but I hadn't realized how complicated they were. I had just gone along with the stories, amused by the clever language and interesting characterizations. Writing this book, I asked myself: Why did Shakespeare complicate his stories to such an extent?

Nowadays, in contrast, most plays are pretty simple in plot and easy to analyze. For instance, *To Kill a Mockingbird* is a powerful stage adaptation by Aaron Sorkin of Harper Lee's 1960 novel. In his version of the story, Mr. Sorkin eliminates the young girl, Scout, as the main character and instead has her father, Atticus, play the role of the main character to simplify the story further. In the stage adaptation, Atticus, a trial attorney and now the protagonist, is representing a Black man, Tom Robinson, who has been accused of rape and the beating of a white woman in 1930s Alabama. The white woman is an abused daughter who has actually been raped by her own father,

Bob. The play explores the widespread racial prejudice rampant in the South at that time. The court rules against Tom, even though Atticus proves that Tom didn't do it.

In Shakespeare, appearance versus reality is a main theme. Elizabethan theater was known for its use of disguises. Shakespeare was no exception, many of his characters conceal their true identities. In this way, they fool other characters but not the audience, who are usually in on the theatrical deception. In *A Midsummer Night's Dream*, appearances confuse the reality of what's happening. There are two worlds in the play: the fairy world and the human world. The fairy world supplies many illusions to the humans. Puck, the main fairy's servant, puts a love potion in the wrong man's eyes, creating more problems. The four lovers in that play are lost and under multiple illusions, as indeed are many lovers in the real world. This underlying theme of appearance versus reality not only amused Shakespeare's audiences, but also caused them to dig deeper into all kinds of meaning in their own lives.

I was reminded of the child's game, peekaboo, the more I thought about why so many illusions and false identities exist in Shakespeare's plays. This game is one in which a player hides her face and then pops back out, to the amusement of the other (usually a baby). Developmental psychologists believe that peekaboo demonstrates a baby's inability to understand object permanence. In cognitive development, the infant achieves the understanding that an object exists, even if the infant is not viewing it, when he or she is about eight or nine months old. Psychologist Jean Piaget did the research to understand this behavior in children.

Shakespeare returns us to childhood and supplies us with sophisticated peekaboo games throughout his plays. Now you think you know a character, but then he changes his identity or he is someone other than who you think he is to begin with. It all results in laughter and delight for the audience.

The Merry Wives of Windsor (1602) is a comedy by Shakespeare that is not considered his best work, although it has been adapted for opera and performed many times. Sir John Falstaff, the portly knight that audiences love, arrives in Windsor without much money. He decides to court two wealthy married women, Mistress Ford and Mistress Page, by sending them identical love letters. He wants his servants, Pistol and Nym, to deliver the love letters. However, the servants refuse, and for this insubordination, they're summarily fired. They go and tell the husbands what Falstaff is planning. Ford is jealous and gets an introduction to Falstaff, calling himself

"Master Brook." Three different men are trying to marry Page's daughter, Anne. She loves Fenton, but the father rejected him because he squandered his considerable fortune. The husband of Mistress Ford, "Master Brook," tells Falstaff he loves her, too, but she's too virtuous to fool around. The wives arrange for a meeting with her and hide Falstaff in a dirty laundry basket. Ford comes back to catch his wife with Falstaff, but the wives, anticipating trouble, have already arranged for the basket with the corpulent knight inside to be dumped into a ditch near the river. Undaunted, Falstaff keeps trying, so the next time he attempts his amorous antics the women disguise him as Mistress Ford's maid's aunt ("the fat woman of Brentford"). He gets beaten up by Ford. The wives eventually tell their husbands the tricks they played on Falstaff. They all devise a last trick—namely telling Falstaff to dress as "Herne the hunter" and meet at an old oak tree in Windsor Forest. Meanwhile, they have the children of the village (including Anne) dress as fairies. They plan to have Anne married off during the festivities. The fairies pinch Falstaff and then reveal their true identities. Falstaff takes all this with good humor. And to complete the hilarious scenario, Anne's two rejected suitors are married off to boys (each man assuming that his "bride" was Anne), while Anne is finally married to the man she truly loves, Fenton. Everyone is forgiven, and the entire entourage has a good laugh about it all.

The themes of the play are sexual jealousy, mistaken identities, revenge, social class, and wealth. At first, I just thought how absurd Falstaff was to go into Windsor and decide to write love letters to two married women there. Was that practice common in Shakespeare's times? And, although we will never know for sure, most likely such a ploy was no more common or acceptable than it is in our own times—albeit with the internet, we now have infinitely more efficient ways of initiating inappropriate and even illicit amorous pursuits. What matters in the world of the theater is the immense power of the absurd. Realizing the utter absurdity of it all causes laughter. What usually makes us laugh is when something or someone is so different from what we're expecting.

I next tried to understand what kind of a personality Falstaff is in the *Merry Wives*. According to many scholars, he's completely different from the way he was in *Henry IV* (parts 1 and 2) and *Henry V* (he does not appear, but his death is dealt with). In *Henry IV*, part 1, the king is disappointed in his son, Hal, who spends all his time drinking and whoring with Falstaff. In *Henry IV*, part 2, Hal redeems himself and rejects Falstaff. Hal becomes king, and when Falstaff tries to reach him, Falstaff is banned.

Some have suggested that Falstaff is just a dramatic device to allow Shakespeare to tell his stories, but I believe he's much more. Falstaff represents our id, the part of us that is wild, aggressive, overtly sexual, and without boundaries. What if we ate and drank whatever we wanted, had sex when we desired it, lied and cheated as we wished? That would be our ids acting out without control, as Falstaff does. In the *Merry Wives*, Falstaff gets his comeuppance with Mistresses Ford and Page playing tricks on him. They represent our mild superegos controlling the id. Sometimes we have to play tricks on ourselves to control our own ids. Master Ford is the punitive superego ready to destroy Falstaff for daring to flirt with his wife. All in all, the audience gets a good laugh with all the mischief and good humor in the play. That explains why we love Falstaff and why he's been represented over and over again in so many stories.

The Merry Wives is Shakespeare's only play not set with aristocrats but with common tradespeople. Also it's the only comedy set in an English town, Windsor.

Henry IV, part 1 (1597), takes off where *Richard II* left off. We are back with the kings and aristocrats. Shakespeare introduces Falstaff in this play to lighten some of the heaviness of serious court drama. King Henry IV faces rebellion from Hotspur, a rash rebellious soldier, and others. Falstaff is a foil for Henry's son, Prince Hal, who is wasting his life with lowlifes. The father fears his son can never become king the way he's going. Henry believes his son is a rebel because he himself was a rebel. He projects his own background onto his son. In the Boar's Head Tavern, Hal and Falstaff and their friends stage imaginary interviews between Henry and Hal. The real interview comes later when Hal promises his father that he will reform himself. Hal kills Hotspur in battle and allows Falstaff to take the credit. Hal later becomes king, and it was through being with Falstaff that he knows about his common subjects.

Henry IV, part 2 (1596), covers the years 1403–1413 and the battle of Shrewsbury with the rebellion of Scroop (archbishop), Hastings, and Mowbray. These three rebels are tricked into abandoning their forces and then executed. Henry IV acts in this way unscrupulously. In part 2, Hal and Falstaff are kept apart, meeting only twice, unlike part 1. This is to show how Hal will evolve into King Henry V. Hal stays at his father's sickbed and is reconciled with him. His father gained his crown through rebellion and so will Hal. Hal identifies with Henry and rejects Falstaff. In psychological terms, he becomes his ego and superego, leaving his id (Falstaff) to be thrown into Fleet Prison.

Troilus and Cressida, probably written in 1602, takes places during the Trojan War. Troilus, a Trojan prince, and Cressida begin a love affair, but Cressida is forced to leave Troy to meet her father in a Greek camp. Once there, Cressida, a Trojan, is exchanged for a Trojan prisoner of war. In the camp, she flirts with Diomedes, and this is observed by Troilus when he attempts to visit her. He vows revenge. The audience is not sure if this play is a comedy or a tragedy, so it has been labeled a problem play. It basically follows the plot of the *Iliad*. Achilles refuses to engage in battle to kill Hector.

While the love story gives the play its name, it accounts for only a small part of the play's focus. The majority of the play revolves around the leaders of the Greek and Trojan forces, Agamemnon and Priam, respectively. Agamemnon, the Greek, and his men attempt to get Achilles to return to battle and face Hector, who sends the Greeks a letter saying he will do one-to-one combat. Ajax is originally chosen to fight, but he makes peace with Hector before they are able to battle. Achilles is prompted to return to battle only after his protégé is killed by Hector before the Trojan walls. A series of skirmishes concludes the play, during which Achilles catches Hector and has the Myrmidons kill him. The conquest of Troy is left unfinished, as the Trojans learn of the death of their hero.

Achilles seems to have narcissistic personality disorder. He refuses to fight in the war and is considered self-centered and grandiose. Although he always needs to win, he considers his pacifism in this war healthy for mankind. He is weak only in his heel, hence the term "Achilles heel," because his mother dipped him in the River Styx to make him powerful. Unfortunately, she held him by his heel, which didn't get into the river. Thus, he was able to be killed by an arrow to his heel.

In *Coriolainus*, written in about 1605, the main character is considered one of Shakespeare's most complex characters. Coriolanus is the name given to a Roman general after his military feats against the Volscians at Corioli. Following his success, he seeks to be a consul (an important Roman magistrate), but his disdain for the peasants and the hostility of the tribunes lead to his banishment from Rome. He presents himself to the Volscians, then leads them against Rome. He suffers from "self-creation fantasies." Coriolainus has been called a schizophrenic, but only by today's standards of analysis. In the play itself, he does not have the sociopolitical viewpoint that he needs to become a warrior because his mother, who played a very influential part in his life, did not teach this to him.

Cymbeline, the Roman Empire's vassal king of Britain, had two sons, Guiderius and Arvirargus, but they were stolen 20 years earlier as infants by an exiled traitor named Belarius. Cymbeline discovers that his only child who is left, his daughter, Imogen, has secretly married her lover Posthumus Leonatus, a member of Cymbeline's court. The lovers have exchanged jewelry. Imogen has a bracelet, and Posthumus has a ring. Cymbeline dismisses the marriage and banishes Posthumus since Imogen—as Cymbeline's only child—must produce a fully royal-blooded heir to succeed to the British throne. In the meantime, Cymbeline's queen is conspiring to have Cloten (her cloddish and arrogant son by an earlier marriage) married to Imogen to secure her bloodline. The queen is also plotting to murder both Imogen and Cymbeline, procuring what she believes to be a deadly poison from the court doctor. The doctor, Cornelius, is suspicious and switches the poison for a harmless sleeping potion. The queen passes the "poison" along to Pisanio, Posthumus's and Imogen's loving servant—the latter is led to believe it is a medicinal drug. No longer able to be with her Posthumus, Imogen secludes herself in her chambers, away from Cloten's aggressive advances.

Posthumus must now live in Italy, where he meets Iachimo, who challenges Posthumus to a bet that he, Iachimo, can seduce Imogen, whom Posthumus has praised for her chastity, and then bring Posthumus proof of Imogen's adultery. If Iachimo wins, he will get Posthumus's token ring. If Posthumus wins, not only Iachimo must pay him but also fight Posthumus in a duel with swords. Iachimo heads to Britain, where he attempts to seduce the faithful Imogen, who rejects him. Iachimo then hides in a chest in Imogen's bedchamber, and, when the princess falls asleep, he emerges to steal her bracelet. He also takes note of the room, as well as the mole on Imogen's partly naked body, to be able to present false evidence to Posthumus that he has seduced his bride. Returning to Italy, Iachimo convinces Posthumus that he has successfully seduced Imogen. In his wrath, Posthumus sends two letters to Britain: one to Imogen, telling her to meet him on the Welsh coast, and the other to the servant Pisanio, ordering him to murder Imogen. However, Pisanio refuses to kill Imogen and reveals to her Posthumus's plot. He has Imogen disguise herself as a boy and continue to the meeting place to seek employment. He also gives her the queen's "poison," believing it will alleviate her psychological distress. In the guise of a boy, Imogen adopts the name Fidele ("faithful").

Back at Cymbeline's court, Cymbeline refuses to pay his British tribute to the Roman ambassador Caius Lucius, and Lucius warns Cymbeline of the

Roman emperor's forthcoming wrath, which will amount to an invasion of Britain by Roman troops. Meanwhile, Cloten learns of the "meeting" between Imogen and Posthumus. Dressing himself enviously in Posthumus's clothes, he decides to go to Wales to kill Posthumus, and then rape, abduct, and marry Imogen. Imogen has now been traveling as Fidele through the Welsh mountains, her health in decline as she comes to a cave: the home of Belarius, along with his "sons" Polydore and Cadwal, whom he raised into great hunters. These two young men are in fact the British princes Guiderius and Arviragus, who themselves do not realize their own origin. The men discover Fidele and, instantly captivated by a strange affinity for "him," become fast friends. Outside the cave, Guiderius is met by Cloten, who throws insults, leading to a sword fight, during which Guiderius beheads Cloten. Meanwhile, Imogen's fragile state worsens, and she takes the poison as a hopeful medicine; when the men re-enter, they find her "dead." They mourn and, after placing Cloten's body beside hers, briefly depart to prepare for the double burial. Imogen awakes to find the headless body and believes it to be Posthumus because the body is wearing Posthumus's clothes. Lucius's Roman soldiers have just arrived in Britain, and, as the army moves through Wales, Lucius discovers the devastated Fidele, who pretends to be a loyal servant grieving for his killed master. Lucius, moved by this faithfulness, enlists Fidele as a pageboy.

The treacherous queen is now wasting away due to the disappearance of her son, Cloten. Meanwhile, despairing of his life, the guilt-ridden Posthumus enlists in the Roman army as they begin their invasion of Britain. Belarius, Guiderius, Arviragus, and Posthumus all help rescue Cymbeline from the Roman onslaught; the king does not yet recognize these four, yet takes notice of them as they go on to fight bravely and even capture the Roman commanders, Lucius and Iachimo, thus winning the day. Posthumus, allowing himself to be captured, and Fidele are imprisoned alongside the true Romans, all of whom await execution. In jail, Posthumus sleeps, while the ghosts of his dead family appear to complain to Jupiter of his grim fate. Jupiter himself then appears in thunder and glory to assure the others that destiny will grant happiness to Posthumus and Britain.

Cornelius arrives in the court to announce that the queen has died suddenly, and that on her deathbed she unrepentantly confessed to villainous schemes against her husband and his throne. Both troubled and relieved at this news, Cymbeline prepares to execute his new prisoners, but pauses when he sees Fidele, whom he finds both beautiful and somehow familiar. Fidele has noticed Posthumus's ring on Iachimo's finger and abruptly demands to know from where the jewel came. A remorseful Iachimo tells of his bet and how he could not seduce Imogen, yet tricked Posthumus into thinking he had. Posthumus then comes forward to confirm Iachimo's story, revealing his identity and acknowledging his wrongfulness in desiring Imogen killed. Ecstatic, Imogen throws herself at Posthumus, who still takes her for a boy and knocks her down. Pisanio then rushes forward to explain that Fidele is Imogen in disguise. Imogen still suspects that Pisanio conspired with the queen to give her the poison. Pisanio sincerely claims innocence, and Cornelius reveals how the poison was a nonfatal potion all along. Insisting that his betrayal years ago was a setup, Belarius makes his own happy confession, revealing Guiderius and Arviragus as Cymbeline's own two long-lost sons. With her brothers restored to their place in the line of inheritance, Imogen is now free to marry Posthumus. An elated Cymbeline pardons Belarius and the Roman prisoners, including Lucius and Iachimo. Lucius calls forth his soothsayer to decipher a prophecy of recent events, which ensures happiness for all. Blaming his manipulative queen for his refusal to pay earlier, Cymbeline now agrees to pay the tribute to the Roman emperor as a gesture of peace between Britain and Rome, and he invites everyone to a great feast.

The character of Cloten represents unrestrained and hypersexuality and bipolarity.

3

Modern Plays

If we're considering modern psychological dramas, we must turn to the plays of Eugene O'Neill (1888–1953). He may be considered a realist inheriting from other great playwrights like Chekhov, Ibsen, and Strindberg, but his plays illustrate so many principles of psychology. He probably suffered from depression and alcoholism—at least many of his characters do.

Anna Christie, one of his plays that won a Pulitzer Prize in 1922, is about Anna, a young woman who is a prostitute. She is idealized by her father, Old Chris, and her boyfriend, Mat, who at first don't realize her profession. The play shows us how we project ideals onto people and how difficult it is to adapt to the reality once we discover it.

Idealization is a primitive defense that employs exaggeration of all-good qualities in an individual and splits off the bad qualities. Idealization satisfies fantasies of unlimited gratification against the reality of frustration with limited gratification that we can obtain from a real, unidealized individual. If we are able to merge the ideal and the real, we begin to mature and understand the world realistically. At the end of *Anna Christie*, Mat and Chris are able to view Anna realistically and forgive her, but then they both leave.

Desire Under the Elms is one of O'Neill's attempts to adapt Greek tragedy to an American story. The myth of Phaedra, Hippolytus, and Theseus is somewhat similar to *Desire Under the Elms*. Phaedra, a Cretan princess and the mother of two sons, falls in love with her stepson, Hippolytus. He rejects her, and she claims she was raped by him to her husband, Theseus. Theseus wants to kill Hippolytus, so he prays to Poseidon, who sends a huge bull or some other monster out of the sea, which scares Hippolytus's horses so that he is dragged to his death. The tragedy ends with Phaedra's suicide. In O'Neill's play, three brothers are dealing with their unresolved feelings about their father. Eben hates his father because he believes his father caused his mother's death, an oedipal emotion played out. Eben's brothers believe that Eben is much like his father. Their father marries a young woman, Abbie, to whom Eben is attracted. She is the new mother that he longs for. Ownership of the farm comes up, and his two brothers leave for California. Abbie promises a son to Eben's father, and then she seduces Eben. It's not clear if it's Eben's son or his father's son who is born. Nevertheless, Abbie kills the child at the end. She then escapes with Eben, even though he called the police on her for the murder of the child.

Mourning Becomes Elektra is a play exploring the theme of revenge and the oedipal complex in women and men. Crimes of the past determine the characters suffering in the present. Critics have compared it to Aeschylus's *Oresteia*. Lavinia, a main character, accuses her mother, Christine, of adultery. Lavinia is then accused by her mother of wanting to steal her place with her husband and her lover Brant. Christine poisons her husband and then accuses Lavinia of the act when Orin, Christine's son, returns. The mother claims her daughter is crazy so Orin will believe her. Lavinia and Orin go abroad and when they return, Lavinia looks like their deceased mother and Orin like their father. Orin reveals that he loves his sister, who is embodying their mother, and then shoots himself. Lavinia throws herself at her mother's lover Brant and then shuts all the windows and throws out all the flowers.

The Iceman Cometh is set in a Greenwich Village saloon and rooming house. There are twelve men and three prostitutes in the play who are alcoholics who spend all their time conning each other and trying to get drinks from the bartender. They all indulge in "pipe dreams," or fantasies. The highlight of their existence is when Hickey, a salesman, shows up and usually buys them drinks. However, when he shows up this time, he is sober and tries to stay that way. For the next four hours, they banter with each other until Hickey reveals that he actually killed his wife. Another character realizes how he tortured his mother, so he kills himself. The "iceman" is like a "milkman" who commits adultery with men's wives. Hickey has killed his wife because he is the one who was unfaithful. The contention of the play is that a person needs a pipe dream to exist. If he gives that up, he is subject to death. In psychoanalytical terms, one needs a defense system against the anxieties of life.

Hughie takes place in the lobby of a seedy Times Square hotel around 1928. There are just two characters: the Night Clerk (Charlie Hughes) and "Erie" Smith, a gambler who occasionally "runs errands" for some of the city's big players. Erie is a small-town hustler who has one long monologue about his bad luck since Hughie died. Hughie is the Night Clerk's predecessor.

Hughie, the former night clerk, is an unseen character whose recent death inspires Erie's long speech on the importance of the patsy.

"Erie"—his nickname is taken from his Pennsylvania hometown—is the big-talking, small-time hustler, a casualty of what remained of the Roaring Twenties before it all crashed.

Erie remembers Hughie's naivete and admiration of Erie's tall tales of gambling and women. Erie hasn't won a bet since Hughie was rushed to the hospital before his death, and now he owes wise guys and old pals the hundred bucks he borrowed to buy a decent floral arrangement for Hughie's funeral. Without Hughie's sympathetic ear listening to his tall tales, Erie is left with the sad truth of his life. Will this new Night Clerk offer a similar escape? Erie has grandiosity and naivete himself to be in this condition. He needs a patsy to project his stories on, and he's hoping the new Night Clerk can accommodate him.

Ah, Wilderness is the only O'Neill play with a happy ending. It's a comedy from 1933 about the Miller family in a small Connecticut town on July 4th. A middle son, Richard, is coming of age as America goes into 1906. He begins to rebel, as is typical of a sixteen-year-old boy, but his loving family supports him and quiets him. Perhaps O'Neill wished he could have originated in such a family or that he could have been that ordinary teenager.

Instead of an ordinary life in a loving family, O'Neill suffered from an unstable family, and in his later years became quite ill from depression and alcoholism. He wanted to write a cycle of eleven plays chronicling an American family, but his health was too poor for him to complete that project. He died in 1953, but he left us more than thirty plays.

If we are considering other playwrights who introduce us to the need for fantasy in people's lives, *M. Butterfly* is certainly worth considering. In *M. Butterfly*, the brilliant contemporary play by David Henry Hwang, Rene Gallimard, a French diplomat in China in the 1950s, falls in love with what he thinks is a beautiful Chinese woman, Song, who is actually a man. He leaves his wife for her and commits espionage against his country. To Gallimard, Song is as beautiful and pure a woman as Madama Butterfly from the eponymous opera. Even when confronted with the truth, Gallimard refuses to dissolve his fantasy about Song. He cannot live without this fantasy, so he dons Song's kimono and puts on her makeup. He becomes his own fantasy.

How much a given defense mechanism contributes to the symptoms and to the ego resistance of a person is what Anna Freud was interested in understanding. She identified and discussed ten defense mechanisms that are commonly recognized in the field of psychoanalysis: regression, repression, reaction-formation, isolation, undoing, projection, introjection, turning against the self, reversal, and sublimation.

The defense mechanisms are not all available to an individual at the same time. As originally proposed by her father, Sigmund, Anna believed that the defense mechanisms developed with the structures of personality (the id, ego, and superego). For example, projection and introjection depend on the differentiation of the ego from the outside world, so they would not be available to the ego as defense mechanisms until the ego had sufficiently developed. This became an important point of contention with analysts like Melanie Klein. Whereas Anna Freud and her colleagues believed that projection and introjection would not be available in early childhood since the structures of personality would not have adequately developed, members of the English psychoanalytical school and Klein believed that projection and introjection were a necessary part of that development. This debate between Freudian and Kleinian theorists continues to this day.

Defense mechanisms are difficult processes to study since much of the processing occurs unconsciously. According to Cramer,[1] as the various fields of psychology developed, they began to examine psychological processes that received new names within the particular field, even though the processes being studied were actually defense mechanisms that had already been discovered within psychoanalysis. For example, what cognitive psychologists describe as selective attention may involve the defenses of splitting and dissociation. In social psychology, scapegoating is a form of displacement. In developmental psychology, when a child's facial expression may be negative while he says something positive it is an example of denial. Therefore, one can conclude that defense mechanisms have remained an important aspect of psychology since they were first described, no matter what school an analyst adheres to.

Susan Glaspell (1876–1948) founded the first modern American theater company, the Provincetown Players, with her husband, George Cook. Her play, *The Verge* (1921), is a psychological study of Claire, who has bipolar disorder. In Act I, she is manic and obsessed with crossbreeding plants. Then she has a compulsion to break with conventional behavior with her first and second husbands and too ordinary daughter. Claire believes she has grown a new species of perverted plant, the "Edge Vine." She retreats to her tower

---

[1] Cramer, P., "Defense Mechanisms in Psychology Today: Further Processes for Adaptation," *American Psychologist*, 55, no. 6 (2000): 637–646.

in Act II and suffers depression. A neurologist goes to treat her. In Act III, she is supposedly rational again, but then strangles Tom, the man she loves. Glaspell wrote three other plays and *Alison's House*, which won the Pulitzer in 1930. *Alison's House* is a biography of Emily Dickinson. The theme is unfulfilled and repressed love that transmutes into poetry.

Trifles (1916), Glaspell's one-act play, shows how women act differently in front of each other versus in front of men. It was written during the first-wave feminist movement. The play begins in an abandoned farmhouse of the Wrights. The county attorney, Mr. Hale, tells how he found Mrs. Wright behaving strangely while her husband was upstairs dead with a rope around his neck. Mrs. Wright said she was asleep when someone strangled her husband. The women downstairs explore the downstairs and find evidence that the wife, who was abused, killed her husband because he killed her pet bird. The men upstairs can't figure anything out, and the women don't tell the men. It's not clear if Mrs. Wright is convicted or not. We are exploring the theme of identity in this play. We never see the Wrights. Glaspell is saying that a person's identity is "constructed" as much as it is innate. Mrs. Wright's identity is only determined by what we hear and see on stage. Silence is powerful in *Trifles*. The women don't speak much; they have a silent solidarity. The men see the women's conversation as trivial. Yet, the women know what happened and the men don't. The women are trapped in their gendered role. They have guilt because they didn't help Mrs. Wright.

Disgraced (2012), by Ayad Akhtar, centers on islamophobia and self-identity. There's a dinner party with four people of different backgrounds: a Muslim lawyer, a Jewish art dealer, an African American, and a WASP artist. Charles Isherwood in the *New York Times*[2] said it "puts contemporary attitudes toward religion under a microscope revealing how tenuous self-image can be for people born into one way of being who have embraced another." The lawyer, Amir, is born in America. He's a merger and acquisitions lawyer who cast aside his Muslim background to get ahead in his career. Emily, his WASP wife, is an artist who focuses on Islamic themes. Amir's nephew, Abe, is worried about a local imam who is jailed because they think he's supporting terrorists. Emily encourages Amir to appear in court to support the imam. Dinner conversation revolves on this case. Is it religious persecution? Amir admits he feels some pride about 9/11 and is hateful toward

---

[2] Isherwood, Charles, "Hottest Tickets of the Year," *New York Times*, December 12, 2012.

Israel. Emily and the art dealer have had an affair in the past to complicate everything.

When I saw *Junk*, a Broadway play by Ayad Akhtar about the 1980s corporate raiders, I started to believe Akhtar was harboring religious prejudice. The protagonist is a Jew whose name, "Merkin," sounds like "Milken," the notorious junk bond trader who went to jail. Since we don't understand his psychology, he remains a stereotype of a greedy Jew. The WASP character, Everson, who owns the steel mill that is being raided, disdains Jews and tries to keep his hold on his business while the Jews invade with junk bonds. Merkin gets in trouble with the feds and is hauled into jail, but not before a lot of anti-Semitic slurs and clichés get thrown around the stage—such as "shylock," "shyster," to mention a few. If this is not prejudice, I don't know what is. And remember, a lot of people think of Jews like this, and, of course, they are convinced that Jews rule the world. One of the only women characters, a journalist who becomes compromised, says right at the beginning that "this is a story about kings."

What bothered me especially was that the playwright, Ayad Akhtar, is not Jewish. It's one thing when Jews joke or criticize their own people, like in the play *Other People's Money* by Jerry Sterner, dealing with the same subject. However, when non-Jewish writers insult and stereotype Jews, it's a completely different story. Akhtar's previous play, *Disgraced*, was also about prejudice. That one dealt with the prejudice against Muslim characters and how they must conform and renounce their religion to fit into Western society. His novel, *American Dervish*, uses characters that express virulent anti-Semitism, although supposedly the novel isn't about that. *Junk* is his first work without Muslim characters, but he really gives it to the Jews in this one. Many movies have addressed this subject as well (e.g., *Wall Street*, *The Big Short*, *The Wolf of Wall Street*, *Equity*), but none of them made me feel there was any anti-Semitic intent, even though they also featured many obviously Jewish characters.

Another contemporary play that addresses prejudice is *A Raisin in the Sun* (1959) by Lorraine Hansberry; it is about a Black family in south Chicago trying to improve their financial situation as they face discrimination. The father, Walter Younger, is barely making a living as a limo driver. He wants to invest in a liquor store with Willy and Bobo, his friends. His (Walter's) father dies, so he will inherit $10,000 with his sister, Beneatha, and their mother. The mother puts some money down on a new house in a white neighborhood because the house is cheaper. She gives Walter $6,500 to invest, but he has to save $3,000 of it for his sister. Willy, his so-called friend, takes the $6,500 and flees instead of investing in a liquor store as they planned. Karl Lindner, a white man from the neighborhood where they want to move, will buy them out because the whites don't want Blacks to live there. Beneatha, Walter's sister, has two boyfriends: George is a fully assimilated Black, and the other, Joseph, from Nigeria, teaches her about African culture. Walter decides not to take the buyout, and in the end, the family is ready to move to the new house in the white neighborhood.

Hansberry captured the mood of the times and also showed us the group dynamics of racial discrimination. One group, the Blacks, are marked as "inferior," while the other group, the whites, are considered "superior." I won't go into American history to discuss how this came about in the United States of America, but in essence, the superior group attempts to keep the inferior group out of their territory. However, this is impossible and against the law, so the conflict escalates. Eventually, the inferior group enters the superior group's domain. We've witnessed how these battles play out all throughout American history. Currently we are still in the midst of it, but we are finally attempting to correct the situation with lectures and courses about systemic racism. The most recent developments to reduce and eradicate racial (and gender) inequality and ethnic injustice include widespread media coverage of racially motivated rioting; new antiracist legislation in Congress; affirmative action employment programs; and ramped-up, nondiscriminatory policies now mandated for public school education and federally funded institutions of higher learning.

Hansberry was unsatisfied with her play, and many considered it too bourgeois. Lorraine Hansberry suffered from depression and had pancreatic cancer, which killed her when she was thirty-four.

Of Mice and Men (1937) is a play adapted from John Steinbeck's novel of the same name. It's about George, a migrant farmworker, and Lennie, a pleasant man with mental deficiencies and a low IQ. Lennie presents as helpless, and George is his savior, who tries to help him stay out of trouble. Lennie, attempting to share his love, results in several deaths of mice, puppies, and eventually a woman. A mob wants to kill Lennie for this, but George kills Lennie first "to put him out of his misery." George and Lennie show the human spirit trying to better itself. They want to save money and buy a ranch. Lennie has a strong erotic attachment to little animals, but he can't control his sadistic impulses toward them. When Lennie and the boss's (Curley's) wife are in the barn together, she invites him to feel her soft hair since he likes to pet soft things. Soon he has his hands around her neck and strangles her to death. George hunts him down before the mob gets there, and while Lennie talks of getting the wished-for ranch and having rabbits, George shoots him. Humans aspiring to peace and security wind up with unconscious impulses that destroy others unless those impulses are acknowledged in psychotherapy.

Our Town (1938) by Thornton Wilder is about a fictional American small town between 1901 and 1913, showing the everyday lives of its citizens. Wilder uses what's called "meta-theatrical" devices, setting the play in the actual theater where it's performed. The stage manager is the main character, and he addresses the audience directly. No props and a mostly bare stage cause the actors to mime actions. In Act I, the stage manager introduces us to the fictional town of Grover's Corners, New Hampshire, and we get the history and meet the characters who go through the day revealing who they are and their conflicts. In Act II, George and Emily reveal their stress as they prepare for marriage. There's an Oedipal moment in this act in which George talks to his mother and says he doesn't want to get old with Emily but with her instead. In Act III, the stage manager talks about eternity as he walks through a cemetery and reveals which characters whom we met at the beginning are now dead. Some deceased characters return to Earth to relive one day. Emily is one of them, who finds it so painful to see that she should have appreciated every day of her life. At least one of these scenes was derived from Freudian concepts.

The Skin of Our Teeth by Wilder (1942) is surrealistic, with one family (the Antrobus's) standing in for all of us. The father is a Freudian figure. In Act I we have the father inventing the wheel because he's in the Ice Age, but he's also in twentieth century New Jersey. Members of the Antrobus family also stand in for biblical characters. In Act II, we're on the boardwalk in New Jersey, where a president is sworn in while a beauty queen tries to seduce him. They go into Noah's ark before Act III, in which the Antrobus family is hiding in a cellar after a war. The theme is that art and literature enhance human life.

Tobacco Road (1933) by Jack Kirkland (adapted from the novel by Erskine Caldwell) shows an economically and psychologically low level of society. One of the characters, Jeeter Lesters, has no suppression of his basic sexual instincts. Father-daughter incest is implied between Jeeter and his girls, Pearl and Ellie May. Sister Bessie, a woman preacher, believes that the Lord gave Ellie May a harelip to keep Jeeter away from her. Pearl, the beautiful one, has a complete abhorrence of sex and doesn't consummate her marriage to Lou.

Many sexually abused women will have this kind of reaction formation when they are finally married. Jeeter and his daughters watch as Jeeter's son, Dude, has sex with Sister Bessie, his wife. Jeeter and his daughters are voyeuristic. Jeeter is so out of it that he has no reactions when the bank takes his farm away or when his wife is killed. This naturalistic drama was all the rage when it was on Broadway because it broke through previous sexual taboos in theater. But many theatregoers were depressed by plays like this because there was no struggle or conflict to rise above their circumstances.

Fleabag (2013) by Phoebe Waller-Bridge is just one long monologue about a young woman's sex life in London, interspersed with how her business partner, Boo, committed suicide and how she had to close up their guinea-pig-themed cafe. It's also the story of her father's rejection of her and her sister after their mother dies from breast cancer.

Sex keeps the play titillating, but it's almost beside the point. We see a very sad young woman who can't mourn her mother or Boo's death. Boo died by suicide after she learned that her boyfriend had sex with another woman. The heroine's father took his daughters to feminist lectures after their mother's death, but then he moved in with the sisters' godmother, and they never saw him again. One night when the heroine is very drunk, she appears at her father's house. He doesn't take her in or care for her. Instead, he gives her cab fare to go home. All the lovers that the heroine has amount to nothing because she can't get her father's love. She is playing out the Electra complex in modern times.

A woman talking freely and passionately about her sex life is still a phenomenon in the United States. We've seen it in stand-up comedy shows by Sarah Silverman and Amy Schumer in our country, but such stories still have the power to shock. In the United Kingdom and Europe, sex tales are more popular than violence stories. A girlfriend of mine from Poland revealed that she watched a lot of sex on TV when she was growing up, but violence on TV was forbidden. Of course, we know the unconscious, the id, is full of sex and violence, and, of course, stage and film artists would tap into these areas for their performances and productions. The different aspects of sex and violence that are permitted or prohibited is fascinating.

The Last Night of Ballyhoo (1996) by Alfred Uhry takes place in Atlanta, Georgia, in 1939. Hitler may have invaded Poland, but the elitist Jews of Atlanta are only concentrating on the social event of the season: Ballyhoo. These are German Jews who have been in America for 150 years. Adolph Freitag, a businessman in his forties lives with his sister, Boo; his sister-in-law,

Reba; and Boo's daughter, Lala. Boo pushes for her daughter Lala to go to Ballyhoo and find a husband. Adolph brings his new assistant, Joe, home with him. Joe is a Brooklyn-born Ashkenazi Jew with ancestors from Eastern Europe. The German Jews of Atlanta look down on Jews like Joe. Joe doesn't want to go to the party with Lala and instead falls in love with Sunny, Reba's daughter, who's home from Wellesley for Christmas. Lala winds up going with Peachy Weiss, who is from a prominent Jewish family. Many events pull the family apart and then pull them back together again.

Alfred Uhry seems to be interested in portraying prejudice, even among Jews who are supposed to be one people.

Uhry is mostly known for *Driving Miss Daisy* (1987)—the first of his "Atlanta trilogy." This play earned him the 1988 Pulitzer Prize for Drama. It shows the relationship between an elderly Southern Jewish woman Daisy and her Black chauffeur, Hoke. Daisy has crashed her car, and her son, Boolie, insists that she hire a driver. Over the next 25 years, Hoke drives Miss Daisy. They argue and are suspicious of each other, but eventually bond. Daisy teaches Hoke to read. When she ends up in a nursing home, it is Hoke who visits her, and she finally confesses to him that he was her best friend. In this play, both main characters are also ultimately involved in the process of overcoming their own individual prejudices: Miss Daisy for Black people and Hoke for white and Jewish people.

There are many more modern plays that I consider in the rest of these chapters. Theater promotes social discourse and social change. We have examined how plays reveal various perspectives, prejudices, psychology of individuals and of groups, and, of course, various psychiatric principles of psychoanalysis.

4

Freud's Contribution

Whenever most people think about psychology or psychiatry, the name Sigmund Freud (1856–1939) comes up. Dr. Freud started his career as a neurologist, but through his work with patients, he discovered and founded psychoanalysis. He is considered the first psychiatrist. The Oedipal complex (see Chapter 1) is a central tenet of his psychoanalytical theory. Many plays illustrate this complex, as it is an essential feature of family dynamics. Free association and transference, as well as the model of the psyche of id, ego, and superego, were elucidated by Freud as well and appear in various plays.

Currently, not many people are able to indulge in psychoanalysis, a treatment in which they lie on a couch four or five times per week, free associate, and feel transference (a projection of feelings from childhood caregivers) to their analyst. However, Freud's theories are a cornerstone of Western thought as well as popular culture. Basically, Freud wanted to make unconscious thoughts conscious. Plays do the same thing in many ways, projecting our unconscious ideas and wishes onto the stage. Our unconscious desires and needs are expressed by the actors. Freud believed that many of his patients in the 1890s had been victims of sexual abuse (his seduction theory). However, since he was already considered bizarre and iconoclastic, he didn't want to completely alienate his peers and the public with his seduction theory, so he suppressed it for the most part. When Jeffrey Masson examined Freud's archives, he discovered that Freud had excised all the case histories dealing with sexual seduction of children. Anna, his daughter, told Masson that her father had abandoned this theory. In his search through Freud's papers, Masson concluded that Freud had suppressed this important theory so that his reputation could be maintained. He should never have done this because the seduction theory takes into account many of the psychiatric problems and patients that we treat to this day.

In Paula Vogel's play, *How I Learned to Drive*, Li'l Bit, the main character, is preyed on by her Uncle Peck from childhood until her twenties. She tells her story backward, so we see her in her adult years suffering from her uncle's sexual abuse. Both she and her uncle turn to alcohol to relieve their anxieties. When I took my medical students to see *How I Learned to Drive* in the theater as part of our "Theater Teaches Psychiatry" program, they were speechless afterward. I tried to encourage them to discuss what we had seen. I said: "Your patients will present with symptoms of addiction, dissociation, depression, somatization. You must learn to recognize that these may be indications that they've been sexually abused. It doesn't matter what medical field you go into." Silence again. Had the subject been declared taboo once again? No, they were only first- and-second-year students—innocent to some extent (and not interested in psychiatry). Freud had swept the issue of child sexual abuse under the rug, too. It is so easy to do even in modern times.

The Greeks were not repressed, so they gave us *Oedipus Rex*. Freud wrote about "the progress of repression" in human life. In his time, real theater and other art forms were blocked by bourgeois morality. His psychoanalysis liberated playwrights and other artists to express raw and true human desires.

Freud wrote sketchy interpretations of *The Merchant of Venice*, *King Lear*, *Richard III*, and *Macbeth*. If Dr. Freud had applied his powerful insights to other plays, that would have been quite enlightening. Nevertheless, his theories provide enough of a basis for us to analyze many works.

Rain (1922), by John Colton and Clemence Randolph, was adapted from Somerset Maugham's story, "Miss Thompson." The fanatic missionary, Reverend Davidson, proselytizes for denial of sex. In psychiatry, his aversion to sex is called "a reaction formation." On their wedding night, he informs his wife that they will have only a spiritual marriage. She becomes frustrated and warped like him as a result of this denial of normal human sexual intercourse. They go to Pago-Pago Island in the South Seas to teach the "pagans." Miss Sadie Thompson, a prostitute, comes to the island, escaping San Francisco and her deeds there. She takes a marine, stationed in Pago-Pago, as a lover. The reverend tries to get her to return to the United States, to prison, but he dreams about mountains that are "like a woman's breasts." The doctor in the play interprets the Davidsons' suppression of sex and contrasts it with the Pago-Pago natives' enjoyment of sex. Reverend Davidson winds up seducing Sadie, and then he kills himself from shame. *Rain* shows how suppressed sexuality is converted into religious fanaticism.

Freud was renowned for exposing the suppressed sexuality of his times. He helped usher in the new realities of playwriting in the 1920s and 1930s, in which playwrights such as Eugene O'Neill and Tennessee Williams broke open conventional beliefs about sexuality.

Theater historians credit Freud and his theories for birthing modern theater. However, Freud's own theater attendance varied throughout his life. In his younger days, he seemed to go frequently, but in later life, he rarely went except to a Mozart opera or Shakespearean play. When writing about plays, he dealt with them as literary products rather than as performances. Did he consider that theater might have a healing, cathartic effect like all art? It seems that Freud was somewhat skeptical about theater's artistic merits, and he was certainly concerned about its emphasis on the irrational. Whatever his personal beliefs were, his ideas had a profound effect on playwrights, such as Schnitzler and O'Neill. Freud's ideas also served as the background for other psychoanalysts interested in the theater, especially Otto Fenichel, who wrote about the actor's personality.

Arthur Schnitzler (1862–1931) was an Austrian playwright and author. He was a contemporary of Freud. Freud supposedly wrote to him and said that Schnitzler learned everything through "intuition," while Freud had to learn everything through "laborious work" on people. Although Schnitzler studied to be a doctor, he abandoned that profession to become an author.

Reigen or *La Ronde* (as it was known by its French name) is a controversial play with provocative sexual themes, written by Schnitzler in 1897. It deals with the sexual and class problems of its day through successive encounters between pairs of sexual partners (before or after sex). Schnitzler shows us characters across all levels of society, and so offers social commentary on how sex transgresses class boundaries. The play was not publicly performed until 1920 in Berlin, Germany, where it provoked strong reactions. Many people called him a pornographer and attacked him for his Judaism.

The scenes are in Vienna in the 1890s with these pairs of lovers:

1. The Whore and the Soldier
2. The Soldier and the Parlor Maid
3. The Parlor Maid and the Young Gentleman
4. The Young Gentleman and the Young Wife
5. The Young Wife and the Husband
6. The Husband and the Little Miss
7. The Little Miss and the Poet
8. The Poet and the Actress
9. The Actress and the Count
10. The Count and the Whore

Schnitzler basically shows us that sexual encounters are the same whether a person is of high class or low, which was scandalous at that time period. Freud of course knew this to be true after psychoanalyzing many patients.

An early play by O'Neill, *Diff'rent* (1920), portrays Emma, a "hysterical" woman with a revulsion for sex. Emma has a "reaction formation," a defense mechanism that is expressed by people presenting with the opposite of their true feelings. This defense is formed because Emma is unconsciously anxious about her real belief. Consciously, she expresses hysteria and revulsion against what she really wants. She breaks off her wedding with her fiancé (Caleb), who had an affair with a native woman in the South Sea Islands. She wants someone "diff'rent" from her father and brother, who both are very sexual. Thirty years later, she's an "old maid" who wants to regress to her youth and seduce a young man (the nephew of her brother), who exploits her for money. Caleb, who's still been celibate for 30 years, loves her, but they don't marry. Instead, they hang themselves at the end.

O'Neill identified himself with Emma, who he saw as an eternal romantic idealist, not as a sexually unfulfilled woman. O'Neill was more interested in Jung than Freud, although now we see a lot of Freudian themes in his early and less successful plays.

There's no single cause for suicide. Suicide most often occurs when stressors and health issues converge to foster hopelessness and despair. Depression is the most common condition associated with suicide, and it is often undiagnosed or untreated. In many plays, suppression of sexuality and other normal feelings lead to suicide. Playwrights do not necessarily show us conditions like depression, anxiety, mania, and substance problems before they have characters commit suicide. Sometimes, they will show us the signs that we psychiatrists look for, such as increased use of alcohol or drugs, a person searching for a way to end his or her life, withdrawing from activities, isolating from family and friends, or giving away prized possessions, like a cat or dog.

In O'Neill's play *The Emperor Jones* (1920), Brutus Jones, a self-assured African American and former Pullman porter, kills another Black man over a dice game. He is jailed but escapes to a backward Caribbean Island, where he sets himself up as emperor. Brutus hacks his way through the jungle to escape former subjects who have rebelled and want revenge against him. Brutus hallucinates as he goes through the forest. These are "racial memories" or connections into a "collective unconscious," which is very Jungian. Jung thought the Oedipus complex, which so interested Freud, was merely the search for the unattainable. To Jung, sexual libido was merely more spiritual energy.[1] In his hallucinations Brutus sees black slaves and a crocodile, which he shoots at the command of a witch doctor.

In *The Hairy Ape* (1922), O'Neill portrays a Yank, Paddy, who loses his sense of belonging on an ocean liner. Since he works below deck, rich people call him a "filthy beast" and exclude him. Paddy regresses to his primitive animal unconscious. He winds up only belonging at the zoo in front of the ape's cage.

The Seagull by Anton Chekhov (1895) is one of his most famous plays and has been analyzed innumerable times.

In act 1, Pyotr, a sick, retired senior civil servant, lives at his country estate. His sister, actress Irina, arrives for a brief vacation with her lover, the writer Boris. Pyotr and his guests view an unconventional play outdoors, which Irina's son, Konstantin, has written and directed. The play-within-a-play features Nina, a young woman who lives nearby, as the "soul of the world" at a time in the future. The play is Konstantin's latest attempt to create something new. Irina laughs at the play, finding it ridiculous. The performance ends prematurely, and Konstantin storms off in humiliation. Irina does not seem concerned about her son. Although others ridicule Konstantin's play, the doctor Yevgeny praises him.

There are many romantic triangles: schoolteacher Semyon loves Masha, the daughter of the estate's steward, Ilya, and his wife, Polina. However, Masha is in love with Konstantin, who is in love with Nina, but Nina falls for Boris. Polina is in an affair with Yevgeny. When Masha tells Yevgeny about her longing for Konstantin, Yevgeny helplessly blames the environment for making everyone feel romantic.

In act 2, a few days later, the characters are outside the estate. Irina argues with the house steward and decides to leave. Nina stays behind, and Konstantin gives her a gull that he shot. Nina is confused and horrified at the gift. Konstantin sees Boris approaching and leaves in a jealous fit.

Nina asks Boris to tell her about the writer's life; he says it's not easy. Nina says that the life of an actress is not easy either, but she wants to be one. Boris sees the gull that Konstantin has shot and muses on how he could use it in a short story: "The plot for the short story: a young girl lives all her life on the

[1] Jung, Gustav, *Psychology of the Unconscious* (New York: Dodd, Mead, 1957). (Original published 1912, trans. 1917.)

shore of a lake. She loves the lake, like a gull, and she's happy and free, like a gull. But a man arrives by chance, and when he sees her, he destroys her, out of sheer boredom. Like this gull." Irina calls for Boris, and she tells him that she has changed her mind—they will not be leaving. Nina lingers behind, enthralled with Boris.

In act 3, Irina and Boris have decided to leave. Konstantin attempted suicide by shooting himself in the head, but the bullet only grazed his head. He spends the majority of act 3 with his scalp heavily bandaged.

Nina finds Boris eating breakfast and gives him a medallion that proclaims her devotion to him. She retreats after begging for one last chance to see Boris before he leaves. Irina appears, followed by Pyotr, whose health has continued to deteriorate. After a brief argument between Irina and Pyotr, he collapses in grief. He is helped off by Semyon. Konstantin enters and asks his mother to change his bandage. She does this, while Konstantin disparages Boris. When Boris reenters, Konstantin leaves in tears.

Boris asks Irina if they can stay at the estate. She convinces him to return to Moscow with her. After she has left the room, Nina comes to say her final goodbye to Boris and to inform him that she is running away to become an actress against her parents' wishes. They kiss and make plans to meet again in Moscow.

Act 4, two years later in the drawing room that is now Konstantin's study, Masha finally accepts the doctor's marriage proposal, and they have a child. Masha still loves Konstantin. Various characters discuss what has happened in the two years that have passed. Nina and Boris lived together in Moscow until he abandoned her and went back to Irina. Nina gave birth to Boris's baby, but it died shortly after birth. Nina never achieved any real success as an actress, and she is currently on a tour of the provinces with a small theater group. Konstantin has had some short stories published, but he is increasingly depressed. Pyotr's health is still bad. People at the estate asked Irina to come back for his final days.

Most of the play's characters go to the drawing room to play a game of bingo. Konstantin does not join them; instead, he is writing. After the group leaves to eat dinner, Konstantin hears someone at the back door. He is surprised to find Nina, whom he invites inside. Nina tells Konstantin about her life over the last two years. Konstantin says that he followed Nina. She starts to compare herself to the gull that Konstantin killed in act 2, then rejects that and says she's an actress but she was forced to tour with a second-rate theater company after the death of her child. Konstantin wants her to stay, but she can't. She embraces Konstantin and leaves. Konstantin spends two minutes silently tearing up his manuscript before leaving the study.

The group re-enters and returns to the bingo game. There is a sudden gunshot from off-stage, and the doctor goes to investigate. He returns and tells Boris to get Irina away because Konstantin has just shot himself.

Freud's Oedipal triangle is quite evident in this play. Konstantin wants his mother's attention, as well as Nina's, but he never gets it because his mother, Irina, and Nina are both entranced by Boris, a father figure. Pyotr, Irina's brother, is another father figure, but he is constantly ailing and not able to assert himself in any way. Because of Konstantin's failure to win his mother or Nina, he kills himself. Suicide happens here because of Konstantin's depression and failure in the Oedipal triangle.

The Seagull has a plot similar to that of *Hamlet*. There is a play within a play. In the same way in which Hamlet tries to win Queen Gertrude back from his uncle, Claudius, Konstantin tries to win his mother from Boris, but he fails. Hamlet fails to win his mother back as well.

The Crucible (1953) by Arthur Miller (1915–2005) ostensibly told the tale of the Salem witch trials in 1692 in Massachusetts. However, Miller wrote the play in the 1950s as an allegory for McCarthyism. At this time in American history, the government persecuted people for either being communists or being suspected of believing in communism. Arthur Miller himself was questioned by the House of Representatives' Committee on Un-American Activities and convicted of contempt of Congress since he didn't reveal the names of colleagues and accuse them of communism or communistic involvements. Miller won the Tony Award for *The Crucible* that year, even though the reviews were not that positive.

The Crucible takes place in a Puritan colony in Salem, Massachusetts. The Reverend Samuel Parris discovered his daughter, Betty, along with Tituba (a slave), and some other girls dancing naked in the forest. Abigail, Samuel's niece, when questioned, denied allegations that the children were engaged in witchcraft. The village is filled with rumors of witchcraft. Actually, the girls were trying to conjure a curse against Elizabeth Proctor. Abigail had had an affair with Elizabeth's husband, John Proctor, when she worked for him as a servant. She was fired for this by Elizabeth. Reverend Hale, a renowned witch hunter, starts to investigate. He accuses Tituba of practicing witchcraft, and she finally breaks down, falsely claiming that the devil caused the problem with her and others. Abigail says that Osborne, Good, and some other women of the town "dance with the devil." Betty accuses other townsfolk.

In act 2, the Proctors mourn the fact that about forty people have been accused of witchcraft. Mary Warren, a servant, gives Elizabeth a "poppet" (a type of doll) and tells the Proctors that people are being hanged. When Hale comes to the Proctors' house, he finds the poppet with a needle stuck in it and accuses Elizabeth of harming Abigail in this way with witchcraft. In response, John submits a deposition signed by ninety-one locals attesting to not only the good character of his wife but also the good repute of some of the other women accused of witchcraft, but the judges dismiss it. Even Reverend Hale (the witch hunter) begins to think this is all ridiculous. John confesses to his affair, but then when his wife is questioned (by herself) she denies it because she doesn't want to incriminate him. The girls and Abigail scream and claim spirits are attacking them. John gives up and says, "God is dead," and they arrest him. There is mass hysteria, and everything and everyone is a mess. Tituba goes insane (hearing voices and talking to Satan). Many villagers are in prison. Twelve were hanged. John does not confess, but he makes up with Elizabeth. At the end, he will be hanged, but he has found his goodness and his cause.

Freud wrote *Group Psychology and the Analysis of the Ego* in 1921. He basically said that when an individual is in a group, he or she acquires infinite power that allows him or her to act on impulses that would otherwise be curbed. The old adage of "safety in numbers" allows the individual to forsake their ego and consciousness and act with the unconscious instead, which leads to violence of every kind. The crowd has a hypnotic effect on the individual and is held together by libidinal bonds.

Freud showed how two groups, the church and the army, for example, can come apart through the loss of libidinal bonds to the leader or among members, and how, in keeping with psychoanalytic dynamics, only the power of love is capable of overcoming the narcissism and hatred that distance us from one another. In *The Crucible*, it is the secret love between Abigail and John Proctor that destroys the entire town. Narcissism is not overcome, and libidinal bonds are destroyed among the townspeople.

Freud identified the psychic formations that ensure group cohesion. He also studied the various known identification processes and distinguished the ego's identifications from those of the ego ideal. He believed: "A primary group . . . is a number of individuals who have put one and the same object in the place of their ego ideal and have consequently identified themselves with one another in their ego" (from the book, *Group Psychology and the Analysis of the Ego* by Sigmund Freud, 1921, International Psychoanalytic Publishing

House). This statement holds true for passionate love and the hypnotic state, which he had used to shed light on the identificatory processes. Freud then verified its validity in the case of the primitive horde, as a structure.

The notion of the intrinsic relationship between individual and group psychology made possible some of his fundamental work on identifications, the ego ideal, and the ego and narcissism. However, the mode of articulation of object relations and identifications remained unknown to him. It would take Klein and others to explain object relations. Freud's ideas about group psychology did not resonate with analysts after him because the majority of psychoanalysts after Freud, when working on groups, have hypothesized Oedipal moments in them.

In *The Crucible*, we see Abigail and the other girls acting as a malignant group to rid themselves of the older people in the village by accusing them of witchcraft. There is hysteria and confusion as they malign their elders. The judges are a group propelled to do harm by these children. Abigail and the other girls are actually the ones that were attempting to do witchcraft, and they project their activities on others. As a group, the young people act with "libidinous impulses," as Freud would say, and then avoid the consequences of their behavior by blaming others. Miller felt the same way about McCarthy and his gang as they falsely accused all of Hollywood of communism.

5

Jungian Concepts

Carl Gustav Jung was a Swiss psychoanalyst who was originally greatly influenced by Freud, who expected Jung to adhere to his points of view. However, Jung broke away from Freud. He rejected the Oedipus complex, and he didn't consider the libido only sexual. He thought of the libido as psychic energy that manifested in three stages of development. Instead, Jung was fascinated by mythology, and not just Greek mythology. Myth for Jung served many functions. First, myth revealed the collective unconscious to the conscious mind; second, dreams for him were analogues of myth. Myth was also a way of thinking, which was the opposite of directed and logical thinking.

Jung thought the lifelong psychological process of differentiation of the self out of each individual's conscious and unconscious elements equals individuation. Jung considered it to be the main task of human development. He created some of the most known psychological concepts. Jung was also an artist, craftsman, and prolific writer, so he was able to use his creativity to formulate many concepts of psychology.

According to Jung, psychoanalysis was to be based on the analysis of dreams, and the analyst had to undergo therapy as well. These were unique concepts in 1912, when Jung proposed them. He was analyzed and then published *Psychological Types*[1] in 1921, contrasting extroversion with introversion. Jung is famous for his "collective unconscious," in which universal archetypes exist. He is known for the concepts of anima versus animus. He described the animus as the unconscious masculine side of a woman, and the anima as the unconscious feminine side of a man. Jung's theory states that the anima and animus are the two primary anthropomorphic archetypes of the unconscious as opposed to the inferior function of the shadow archetypes. He believed they are the abstract symbol sets that formulate the archetype of the Self.

[1] Jung, Carl, *Psychological Types* (1934; repr., Princeton, NJ: Princeton University Press, 1976).

In Jung's theory, the anima makes up the totality of the unconscious feminine psychological qualities that a man possesses and the animus the masculine ones possessed by a woman. Jung believed a man's sensitivity is often lesser or repressed, and therefore considered the anima one of the most significant features. The anima and animus manifest themselves by appearing in dreams and influence a person's attitudes and interactions with the opposite sex.

Synchronicity describes circumstances that appear meaningfully related yet lack a causal connection. In contemporary research, synchronicity experiences refer to a person's subjective experiences that coincide between events in their mind and the outside world that may be causally unrelated to each other yet have some other unknown connection. Jung held that this was a healthy, even necessary, function of the human mind that can become harmful.

Jung also gave us the principle of opposites, in which every wish immediately suggests its opposite. According to Jung, it is the opposition that creates the power or libido of the psyche.

The attitudes and functions operate as pairs of opposite and compensatory tendencies. According to Jung, whichever attitude or function dominates consciousness, its opposite will tend to be repressed and to characterize the compensatory activity of the unconscious.

Opposites are, psychologically, the ego and the unconscious. There is no form of human tragedy that does not in some measure proceed from the conflict between the ego and the unconscious.

Jung described various archetypes that he considered fundamental to the psychological makeup of every individual: the mother, the child, the shadow, the father, spirit, and trickster. Archetypes are archaic forms of innate human knowledge passed down from our ancestors.

In Jungian psychology, the archetypes represent universal patterns and images that are part of the collective unconscious. Jung believed that we inherit these archetypes in much the same way we inherit instinctive patterns of behavior.

He distinguished two general attitudes (introversion and extraversion) and four functions: thinking, feeling, sensing, and intuiting.

Applying Jungian concepts to play analysis reveals many unique ideas. August Strindberg was a Swedish playwright who developed new forms of dramatic action, language, and visual composition. The play *Miss Julie* opens with Jean, the valet, coming on the stage, which is set in the kitchen of the manor. He talks to Christine, a maid, about Miss Julie's strange behavior. He wants to open an inn with Christine. Miss Julie went to the barn dance and tried to dance with him and the gamekeeper. Everyone was shocked. Jean and Christine are engaged to be married, but that didn't stop Miss Julie from flirting with Jean. She enters the kitchen and demands that Jean waltz with her in front of Christine. He tries to refuse, but Miss Julie insists. Eventually, they wind up in Miss Julie's room and have sex. Then they want to run off together, but Miss Julie realizes that she has no money. At the end, Jean hands her a razor, with the implication that she should kill herself.

Jung would consider Miss Julie an extroverted character, that is, talkative, energetic, concentrating on the external "object," in this case Jean. Miss Julie seeks gratification outside of herself. In Jung's world, if she were introverted, she would be more reserved and reflective and take pleasure in solitary activities. Her extroversion gets her into trouble. In 1888, when Strindberg wrote the play, the upper classes didn't mix with the lower classes so easily, and when they did, disaster ensued.

The Dance of Death, parts 1 and 2, was also written by Strindberg. The story is about a husband and wife who hate each other, who are vicious and sadistic toward each other, but are trapped in their miserable marriage. They will be celebrating their twenty-fifth wedding anniversary. The husband, Edgar, is a retired artillery captain and a tyrant. The wife, Alice, is a former actress. They live isolated on an island and are not popular or social. Their children do not live with them; each parent has turned the children against the other parent. Edgar has heart problems and may not have long to live. Alice sometimes plays the piano as her husband dances a kind of bizarre saber dance. As he dances, she hopes it might kill him, and he threatens to cut her out of his will.

The third important character is Kurt, who is Alice's cousin. He visits and learns that in the past the captain worked with Kurt's former wife in a way that caused Kurt to lose custody of his own children in his divorce. Kurt and Alice join forces to plot against her husband, and the cousins' relationship becomes passionate and sexual, as Alice wants him to kiss her foot, while Kurt talks of bondage and bites her like a vampire. "Vampire" and "cannibal" are significant images in this play and are used against the captain. Jung would say the cousins are playing out archetypal and mythological roles. Their libidos are enhanced with these images.

The story paves dark passages into the human mind. In the final moment, what has survived amid the emotional and psychological wreckage is, unexpectedly, the marriage. The play ends right where it started.

Hedda Gabler (1891) by Henrik Ibsen, a Norwegian playwright, focuses on Hedda, the daughter of a general, trapped in a marriage and house that she doesn't want. This story reveals a depraved society sacrificing its citizens' freedom and individual expression. Hedda is narcissistic enough to pursue what she wants, but she is also afraid of breaking the rules. She's torn between these two states. She may face public scandal, but decides to kill herself to escape this fate. Ibsen also investigated the subject of women trapped in his world in *A Doll's House*. *Hedda Gabler* takes Ibsen's analysis further. Hedda is a modern Medea, who defines herself negatively, destroying what she can't accept. Nora, in *A Doll's House*, left her husband and children and went to find herself. Hedda cannot do that, so she focuses her rage on herself. Hedda's libido is powerful, not only sexually but also psychically. Jung believed psychic energy could be channeled externally (toward the world) or internally (toward the self). Hedda does both: She channels her energy toward men who are lovers, and then she channels internally and, in her case, into self-hatred. Jung proposed three basic principles of the psychic energy: (1) opposites; (2) equivalence; (3) entropy.[2] Jung would not consider Hedda just sexually frustrated as Freud would have. From Jung's viewpoint, Hedda was motivated intellectually and creatively, but she wasn't educated enough to express herself, so her intelligence and psychic energy became stultified. She derived some vicarious pleasure through Lovborg's work but could never satisfy her needs.

Jung was also interested in male psyches and homosexuality. He believed that a son's "mother complex" leads to self-castration, madness, and early death. He also thought that the effects on the son are homosexuality and Don Juan-ism and impotence.[3]

A famous mother who Jung wrote about was Cybele, who was originally introduced in Anatolia (an ancient country in Asia Minor). She was known as the mother of all gods and of all life and came to be regarded as a protectress of civilization. Cybele is connected to lions and hawks. The mythology is that she fell in love with a handsome shepherd, Attis, but he was in love with

[2] Symbols of Transformation (Collected Works of C.G. Jung, Volume 5) by C.G. Jung, Princeton University Press; 2nd edition, 1977.
[3] Jung, Carl, *The Basic Writings of Jung* (New York: Modern Library, 1959).

a nymph, Sagaris. When Attis and Sagaris had a wedding, Cybele crashed the wedding. When she appeared, she scared Attis so badly that he fell at the base of a pine tree while climbing in the mountains. In his madness, he mutilated himself and bled to death there. Pine trees then became sacred when Jupiter and Cybele blessed them in honor of Attis.

The mother is the first feminine being that the son encounters usually. The son identifies or resists identification with the mother; there's a constant attraction and repulsion going on. Jung thought that if this ambiguity is not resolved, the son becomes gay.

Angels in America, Part 1: Millennium Approaches (1991) and *Part 2: Perestroika* by Tony Kushner won a Pulitzer Prize, a Tony, and a Drama Desk Award for an Outstanding Play. It is a complex examination of homosexuality and AIDS in America in the 1980s. There are angels and ghosts and all sorts of metaphorical characters. Jung would have been delighted by the symbolism. The play starts with the funeral of Louis's grandmother Sarah. The main mother, Sarah, has died, so the boys can play, since they are no longer encumbered by feminine authority. Louis learns that his lover, Prior Walter, has AIDS. Louis abandons him, but an ex–drag queen nurse, Belize, cares for Prior. The gay community creates their own mothers to help them. Joe Pitt, a Mormon Republican clerk who is secretly gay, begins an affair with Louis. Joe's wife, Harper, is a weak woman addicted to Valium. Harper is so out of it that she thinks she's in Antarctica while wandering the streets of Brooklyn. Women are seen as weak and inadequate in this play. Roy Cohen, who is advising Joe, has AIDS, which he lies about. Roy sees the ghost of Ethel Rosenberg, whom he had executed for espionage. A woman is only safe in this play if she's a ghost, weak, or a female angel, the most powerful and unrealistic woman.

In part 2, Prior is told by the angel that Heaven is like San Francisco, and that after the San Francisco earthquake of 1906, God abandoned Heaven. Humans must stop moving so that Heaven and God will be restored. Roy winds up in the hospital, too, and steals the AZT (zidovudine) supply, with Belize caring for him and Ethel's ghost helping or not helping. Joe and Louis break up because of Joe's hypocrisy about his gayness and his connection to Roy Cohen. Roy sees Ethel as his mother before he dies. Louis and Belize steal Roy's supply of AZT for Prior. Prior wrestles the angel, who then opens a ladder into Heaven for him. It was a fever dream, and then he wakes up in the hospital. The play ends in 1990. Prior's mother, Hannah, accepts her son as he is. The gay son's final acceptance from a mother ends the ambiguity that is such a struggle with gay men and their mothers.

Jung's interpretation of dreams consisted of finding archetypes and symbols with which the unconscious supplied the conscious.[4] The same holds true for August Strindberg's *A Dream Play* (1901). In this play, Agnes, a daughter of the Vedic god Indra, descends to earth to bear witness to human problems. She meets 40 characters (some of which are symbols of theology, philosophy, medicine, and law). After experiencing all kinds of human suffering, Agnes realizes we humans are to be pitied. Then she wakes up when she returns to heaven. Strindberg said he gave up his cause-and-effect plays to write this one. He followed associative links like those found in a dream. The dreamer's consciousness rules the play. Things split, dissolve, and merge in a dream-like way. It is believed that Strindberg wrote *A Dream Play* after experiencing a psychotic break in which he thought witches wanted to murder him.

A Midsummer Night's Dream by Shakespeare (1595) is famous for being a play that contains other plays within it, as well as many subplots. Theseus, duke of Athens, is about to marry Hippolyta, queen of the Amazons, who thinks she is dreaming. They are visited by Egeus; his daughter, Hermia; and two of her suitors. Egeus complains that Hermia won't marry Demetrius, his choice of the suitors. By Athenian law, she can be put to death for not obeying her father, but she loves Lysander. The duke agrees with Egeus. Hermia and Lysander meet secretly and agree to leave Athens and go marry in another town. Helena, who loves Demetrius, finds out about the elopement and tells Demetrius. They go after the lovers. Another subplot involves a group of six amateur actors—Quince, Bottom (plays Pyramus), Flute, Starveling, Snout, and Snug—rehearsing a play they are supposed to perform for Theseus before his wedding. Everyone winds up in a forest with Machiavellian fairies, who manipulate the humans. The fairies (Oberon, Titania, and Puck) make the wrong humans fall in love with each other through a magic potion applied to the eyelids. They turn Bottom's head into that of a jackass. Since the humans can't phantom what the fairies are doing, they all decide they are dreaming. In the play within the play, Pyramus and Thisbe are lovers who have eloped just like Hermia and Lysander. The amateur actors do a terrible job, but there's a happy ending when Theseus arranges a group wedding.

Major Barbara (1905) by George Bernard Shaw shows us Barbara Undershaft, an idealistic young woman, who helps the poor in the Salvation Army in London. Her father, Mr. Undershaft, is a successful and wealthy

---

[4] Jung, Carl, *Dreams* (Princeton, NJ: Princeton University Press, 1974).

businessman making guns, submarines, and battleships in his munitions factory. He is separated from Barbara's mother, Lady Britomart Undershaft. Lady Britomart wants to get money for Barbara and her other daughter, Sarah. Barbara hasn't seen her father since she was little. Mr. Undershaft comes over to see his children and agrees to visit the Salvation Army shelter if Barbara will visit his factory afterward. Mr. Undershaft is impressed with the shelter and the way his daughter handles the fractious people who are there receiving help. She is sincere and patient, even though the people receiving social services are difficult. Mr. Undershaft decides to make a big donation to the Salvation Army, but his daughter doesn't want to accept it because it comes from armaments and alcohol. Barbara's supervisor grabs the offer of money, so Barbara is left disillusioned. Mr. Undershaft has to leave his fortune to a foundling by tradition. It turns out Cusins, a scholar and Barbara's fiancé, is a foundling who can marry Barbara. She has to overcome her horror of her father's money. Mr. Undershaft declares he's doing more good work than Barbara since he employs many workers.

Shaw often has the innocent women in his plays become disillusioned and brought down to earth by the reality of situations. He did this in his play *Arms and the Man*, and he does this in this play with Barbara. In *Saint Joan*, Joan of Arc never comes down to earth. She always is idealistic, which allows her to win her battles. In Jungian terms, Shaw's heroines are archetypical mothers.

Blithe Spirit (1941), by Noël Coward, is a favorite play of many theaters. I've seen it often, from Broadway to Los Angeles. The socialite, Charles, invites a medium and clairvoyant, Madame Arcati, to his house so they can have a séance. Charles is a novelist, and he hopes to get material for his next novel. However, Madame conjures up Charles's deceased first wife. Elvira was annoying, and her ghost still is. She tries to disrupt the relationship with his present wife, Ruth, who is oblivious to Elvira as only Charles can see and hear her.

The title, *Blithe Spirit*, is taken from a Percy Bysshe Shelley poem, "To a Skylark."

Ruth is a conventional woman who doesn't believe in ghosts until (an invisible) Elvira hands her a vase out of thin air. Elvira sabotages Charles's car, hoping to kill him so he can join her in the spirit world.

However, it's Ruth who is killed instead of Charles. Ruth comes back as a ghost to revenge herself on Elvira. Charles can't see Ruth, but he sees Elvira running around causing chaos because Ruth is chasing her. Madame Arcati comes back to exorcise both spirits, but she only manages to materialize Ruth.

Madame goes through many séances trying to get rid of them. She can't until she realizes that the maid is the conduit that the spirits are coming through. Madame tells Charles to leave, even though she has made the two ghosts invisible since they may still be there. Charles tiptoes out, and the two unseen ghosts wreck his house.

Jung was open to ghosts from an early age. When he visited Britain, he stayed in a country cottage that was haunted by a ghost, an old woman with half her face gone. His psychology lent itself to unseen worlds and other dimensions. His conceptions of intuitions fit in with dealing with the spiritual world. Jung believed we couldn't use two perceptual functions at the same time. We can only use one at a time. So Ruth (when she was living) couldn't use her intuition to see Elvira. She was too much of what Jung would call the "thinking" type—the type that loves logic and rationality. Charles could see Elvira because he was an intuitive writer.

6

Adlerian Complexes

Alfred Adler (1870–1937) is often categorized under psychoanalysis with Freud and Jung. However, this is not accurate. Dr. Adler was more of a Gestalt psychiatrist and an advocate of the individual, although he also considered the person in relation to the social environment. He wrote about the aggression drive, the neurotic disposition, and masculine protest. According to Adler, the neurotic person lacks confidence, is oversensitive, guilty, and inhibits aggression. Adler's most famous book is *The Neurotic Constitution*.[1]

Dr. Adler introduced his theories of individual psychology with this book. He made it clear that consciousness and unconsciousness both serve the individual in a consistent life plan. The term *inferiority complex* comes from Adler's theory of personality.

Masculine protest is a concept described by Adler. In women, it gives expression to a rejection of their feminine condition, the consequence of a devaluation of girls in their family or cultural milieu and the choice of a masculine ideal in the formation of their guiding principle. In men, it expresses itself as a superiority complex and striving to dominate.

Adler wrote[2]: "When a girl imagines that she can change into a boy, it is because the feminine role has not been presented to her as the equal of the masculine role. She revolts against what she believes to be a permanent perspective of inferiority for her. The Freudians have interpreted this fact as what they call the 'castration complex.'" This rejection of the feminine role is also the consequence of the mother's preference for her son or sons, which constitutes a paradox. Writing about one of his patients, Adler said: "Her mother, a fact that is unfortunately very frequent, had more affection for her sons than for her daughter, which confirms that she also accorded greater value to the male principle without, however, giving her husband the advantage that is inherent in this mode of appreciation." This withdrawal of libido

---

[1] Adler, Alfred, *The Neurotic Constitution* (millionbooks, 2003). (Original from Moffat, Yard and Company, New York, 1917.)

[2] Adler, Alfred, *Social Interest: A Challenge to Mankind* (Germany, 1938). One World, UK, 1998.

from the father facilitates father-daughter alliances. This patient had become the boss of the house. Speaking of another patient, he commented: "In her childhood antecedents we find a powerful feeling of inferiority, maintained in a constant state of tension by the fact that her mother preferred her younger brother and that he was more intelligent than she was. This patient's most ardent conscious desire was always to be tall, very intelligent, to be a man."

A conflictual relationship with the mother exaggerates the need to compensate against the inferiority complex through the elaboration of an ideal model and leads to a hostile attitude to women. Sexual and aggressive instincts then come together either in masculine behavior that rivals with men or in homosexual behavior where a dominant role is assumed. When the woman becomes a mother herself, she can transpose these problems to her relations with her children. Nowadays when it is possible to have a sex change, women transcend their roles and become masculine to their fullest fantasies. Adler would have to establish new theories to explain our present transitions.

Tennessee Williams (1911–1983) was an American playwright whose real name was Thomas Lanier Williams III. He, along with Eugene O'Neill and Arthur Miller, is considered one of the greatest American twentieth-century playwrights. He gave us *The Glass Menagerie*, *A Streetcar Named Desire*, *Cat on a Hot Tin Roof*, *Sweet Bird of Youth*, *The Night of the Iguana*, and *The Rose Tattoo*, just to mention a few of the most famous ones. He wrote over 70 one-act plays in addition to his full-length ones. In many of his works, Williams was dealing with his homosexuality, which had to be kept in the closet during that time period. He struggled with masculine protest of a different sort.

In *The Glass Menagerie*, Tom, the narrator, feels totally inferior because of the way his mother treats him and the fact that he has to work at a shoe factory to support the family. He runs away from his autistic sister, Laura Wingfield, and escapes through literature and alcohol. In *A Streetcar Named Desire*, Stanley Kowalski has an inferiority complex and that's why he is abusive and rapes his wife's sister, Blanche Dubois, who "relies on the kindness of strangers." In *M. Butterfly*, by David Henry Hwang, the main character, Gallimard, has an inferiority complex in desiring the perfect woman, who in fact is a man.

Adler believed that Freud emphasized sex too much as a primary cause of neurosis. He stated that sex was a symptom of neurosis as well as a cause. He was more interested in individuals striving for superiority because they feel inferior. The will-to-power or aggression is important in his studies. Dr. Adler actually contributed more to the psychology of parent-child relationships than Freud did. He also used Gestalt psychology, which emphasizes the patterns that humans perceive, rather than individual components. *Gestalt* is a German word that means pattern or configuration. Max Wertheimer, Kurt Koffka, and Wolfgang Koehler founded Gestalt psychology in the early twentieth century. They were intent on not breaking psychological phenomena into its basic elements or atoms. Instead, they wanted to view the whole or entire structure or consciousness as structure.

Awake and Sing (1935) by Clifford Odets is a great example of a playwright using psychological patterns to tell his stories. All his characters are struggling for life among lowly conditions. The mother, Bessie Berger, serves as both mother and father to her Bronx family since the father, Myron, is a passive-aggressive dependent little man. Ralph, their son, feels quite inferior since he had such a terrible childhood. Ralph has a girlfriend, but Bessie, his mother, opposes her with Oedipal jealousy. Ralph's sister, Hennie, gets pregnant, and Bessie decides Hennie should marry the neurotic Sam since they can't find the man who impregnated Hennie. Jacob, the old grandfather, tells the family to awake and sing. Then he jumps off the roof. He leaves his money to Ralph, which makes Ralph mature into a man. The Berger family is eloquent in their inferiority feelings.

Cock (2009) by Mike Bartlett is about a gay man, John, who is in a relationship with his boyfriend, M., for seven years. John meets and falls in love with W., a woman. John tells M. about it. The last scene is supposed to be like a cock fight, in which M. and W. fight about who will get John. Dr. Adler would say that both John and M. suffered from inferiority complexes, and they were exhibiting masculine protest. The aggression drive is clearly illustrated as well.

Adler felt that "masculine protest" was a striving for dominance that men engaged in with each other. He fought the concept of "the real man," which was prominent in his time. He broke away from Freud because he believed the aggression drive was more than biological.

Glengarry Glen Ross (1984), a play by David Mamet, shows how desperate real estate agents are to sell their undesirable properties. The men compete with one another for "leads" (names and phone numbers of potential clients). They are ready to steal, intimidate, bribe, and threaten each other. They exhibit masculine protest and aggression in a "dog-eat-dog environment."

Women who refuse to do anything they consider feminine are also exhibiting "masculine protest." The woman could be a police officer, firefighter, or truck driver, or any job traditionally considered masculine. Both the women and the men described in *Glengarry Glen Ross* are attempting to gain power and dominance in a particular situation. Dr. Adler theorized that they needed power because of their feelings of inferiority. Women are often portrayed as strong and dynamic figures in Greek drama (e.g., *Agamemnon*, *Antigone*, *Medea*, *Lysistrata*; see Chapter 1), but in ancient Greek society most women were considered less than second-class citizens and basically confined to their homes. According to Adler, these exceptional women portrayed in Greek drama were engaging in masculine protest.

Adler had a distinctive approach to trauma as an occurrence that decreased a person's connection to society—a concept that he considered extremely important for meeting life's tasks. Trauma increases feelings of inferiority and inadequacy. We see all kinds of trauma in Greek drama—trauma that leads to murder and violence. And in *Glengarry Glen Ross*, the trauma of the characters is pulsating just below the surface as the characters struggle for survival.

Adler thought of dreams as infantile claims to power. He felt that dreams, daydreams, and fantasies all expressed an individual's lifestyle. Although Adler admitted that dreams serve a problem-solving function, he also felt that he solved his own problems in waking life and so claimed never to dream.

Miss Firecracker Contest by Beth Henley (1984) is set in a small southern town where all the characters feel inadequate and strive to be accepted. Carnelle, the main character, is a young woman in her twenties striving to repair her reputation as "Miss Hot Tamale." She's dealing with her two cousins, Elain and Delmount. The cousins' mother, Carnelle's aunt, has died of a pituitary gland cancer. They gave the aunt a monkey's gland, which didn't work to save her, but instead made her grow long black hair on her body. Carnelle is an orphan who was taken in by her aunt. Elain is beautiful, married with two kids, and escaping her husband. Delmount was just discharged from a mental hospital. Carnelle gave Mac Sam, a boyfriend, syphilis, and he already had tuberculosis and a bad liver. Carnelle constantly feels inadequate as she practices for the "Miss Firecracker" contest. Her friend, Popeye (a seamstress), falls in love with Delmount from his picture, even before he comes on stage. All the characters are unique and believable as inhabitants of a small southern town struggling to find their places in the world. Carnell only comes in fifth place in the contest. She has a wonderful costume sewn by Popeye.

The Homecoming (1964) by Harold Pinter is about Teddy and Ruth's "homecoming." Teddy is a philosophy professor in the United States. Ruth is Teddy's wife. They have lived in the United States for six years. Ruth has never met her husband's working-class family in North London, where he grew up. They married in London before going to the States. Ruth teases Teddy's brothers (Lenny, a pimp; and Joey, a boxer); as well as his other close male relatives (Sam, Teddy's uncle; and Max, Teddy's father). In act 1, Max (the patriarch of the whole family and Teddy's father) is struggling for dominance with Lenny. They imply that Sam is gay and insult the other men in the family. Teddy and Ruth arrive and talk about their three sons in the Unites States. The couple is having problems. Ruth flirts with her brother-in-law Lenny and then leaves. The next morning when Ruth and Teddy are present, Max assumes Ruth is a prostitute because no one told him the couple had arrived the night before. Teddy reconciles with Max. In act 2, the men all light cigars in a family masculine ritual. Max reminisces about his late wife, his job as a butcher, and his boys. Ruth was a "photographic model for the body." Teddy goes upstairs to pack. He wants to get back to the United States quickly. When he returns, Ruth and Lenny are slow dancing. Then Ruth and Lenny kiss with everyone watching. Lenny turns her over to Joey, Teddy's other brother, saying: "She's wide open." Joey makes out with her. Max says that next time Teddy should tell him if he's married or not and that he understands Teddy is ashamed of a woman "beneath him." Ruth pushes Joey away and takes command suddenly, but she goes upstairs with Joey. He comes back later and says she refused to go "the whole hog." The men downstairs brag about their sexuality. When Ruth comes downstairs, Teddy gives her a proposition to be a prostitute, and she announces her terms: a three-room flat and a maid. She wants a signed legal document. Sam collapses on the floor and is presumed dead by the family. Teddy leaves without Ruth, and she is left sitting as if on a throne with the men. When I saw the play, I was amazed that Teddy did not try to defend Ruth against his family. Instead, he pimps her out to them.

Is the "homecoming" Ruth's, not Teddy's? Has she rediscovered her previous identity as a prostitute? She is the only woman in a play of men. Dr. Adler would say that the men are striving for dominance over each other, but the woman Ruth wins in the end. She is the mother/wife/whore. Teddy has been in denial about her previous life and just viewing her as the wife and mother of his three sons.

Pinter often wrote in an ambiguous way and didn't have a set plot resolution at the end of his plays. His characters are forceful and significant in their actions more than in their words. He is the master of minimalism, and he challenges the set morals of this times. Psychologically, women are seen in this trilogy of mother/wife/whore by men. Pinter lays it out in this often-puzzling play.

The Caretaker (1960) by Pinter is a study of power and allegiance also. Two brothers and a tramp are the main characters. In act 1, Aston has invited Davies, a homeless man, into his apartment after he rescued him from a bar fight. The homeless man is critical of the apartment. Aston gives him shoes to try on, but he doesn't like any of them. They go to sleep, but Davies keeps Aston up all night with his muttering. Davies says he's not doing that. Aston leaves, and Davies goes through his stuff. Mick, Aston's brother, arrives and sneaks up on Davies and fights him. In act 2, Mick demands Davies's name. Davies claims he can establish his identity if he gets papers in Sidcup. Aston returns with a bag, and they all fight over that. Aston offers Davies a job as caretaker of the flat, but Davies fears taking the position. The next day, Aston reveals he was in a mental hospital getting electroshock therapy, which left him "brain damaged." Davies wants to throw Aston out and take over the place. He tries to conspire with Mick, but eventually the two brothers bond and kick Davies out. Dr. Adler would interpret this behavior as men competing with each other once again.

True West (1980) by Sam Shepard is the classic story of sibling rivalry between two brothers, Austin and Lee. They're in their mother's house and just meeting again after five years. Lee is older and more dominant than Austin. Their mother is on vacation in Alaska. Austin is house-sitting and trying to work on his screenplay. Lee distracts him with silly questions. Lee wants to steal things from the neighborhood, and he's concerned about the security of their own house. Austin wants Lee to leave because Saul, a film producer, is coming over. Lee leaves, but he demands Austin's car keys for the favor of leaving. Saul and Austin are discussing an agreement when Lee comes back with a stolen TV. Surprisingly, Saul and Lee talk about golf and make plans to play the next day. Austin is excluded, and Austin has to type Lee's story that he will present to Saul. In act 2, Lee returns with the golf clubs Saul gave him as an advance on his story. Austin is supposed to write up Lee's idea since Saul is dropping Austin's screenplay. When Saul is confronted, he wants Austin to write both his and Lee's story, but Austin refuses. Saul drops Austin and wants to get another writer for Lee's story. Austin gets drunk and annoys Lee, who is typing up his screenplay. They fight and then make a deal that Austin will write the play for Lee if Lee takes him to the desert. Finally, the house is a mess, and the two brothers are working on the script when their mother returns home. Their mother is astonished by what she sees. She storms out. The brothers fight, and Austin almost kills Lee. The play ends.

Again, Dr. Adler would say these two brothers are competing and struggling for dominance. Each feels inferior in his own way. Austin is the younger and attempting to break into the film world. The older brother, Lee, has abandoned society; he's a proud thief. Amazingly enough, Saul prefers his idea to Austin's script.

In *The Winter's Tale* (1623) by William Shakespeare, Leontes, the king of Sicily, is entertaining Polixenes, the king of Bohemia, in his kingdom. They are old friends, but after nine months, Polixenes wants to return to his own kingdom to tend to affairs and see his son. Leontes wants Polixenes to stay longer, but he can't convince Polixenes. Leontes then sends his wife, Queen Hermione, to convince Polixenes. Hermione agrees, and she is soon successful. Leontes is puzzled about how Hermione convinced Polixenes so fast, so he begins to suspect that his pregnant wife has been having an affair with Polixenes and that the child is Polixenes'. Leontes orders Camillo, a Sicilian lord, to poison Polixenes. Camillo instead warns Polixenes, and they both flee to Bohemia.

Leontes is incensed at their escape, and he publicly accuses his wife of infidelity. Also, he says that the child she is bearing is illegitimate. He throws her in prison over the protests of his nobles and sends two of his lords, Cleomenes and Dion, to the Oracle at Delphos for what he is sure will be confirmation of his suspicions. Meanwhile, the queen gives birth to a girl, and her loyal friend Paulina takes the baby to the king to soften his heart. He's paranoid and grows angrier, however, and orders Paulina's husband, Lord Antigonus, to take the child and abandon it in a desolate place. Cleomenes and Dion return from Delphos with word from the Oracle. Hermione claims to be innocent and asks for the words of the Oracle to be read before the court. The Oracle states that Hermione and Polixenes are innocent. Further, the oracle says Camillo is an honest man, and that Leontes will have no heir until his lost daughter is found. Leontes refuses to give up his delusion and believe that this is the truth. As this news is revealed, word comes that Leontes's son, Mamillius, has died of a wasting sickness brought on by the accusations against his mother. At this, Hermione falls into a coma and is carried away by Paulina, who subsequently reports to her heartbroken husband that the queen is dead. Leontes vows to spend the rest of his days atoning for the loss of his son, his abandoned daughter, and his queen.

Antigonus, meanwhile, abandons the baby on the coast of Bohemia, reporting that Hermione appeared to him in a dream and asked him to name the girl Perdita. He leaves a bundle of gold and other trinkets by the baby to show that the baby is of noble blood. A violent storm suddenly appears, wrecking the ship on which Antigonus arrived. He wishes to take pity on the child but is chased away by a bear. Perdita is rescued by a shepherd and his son. "Time" enters and announces the passage of sixteen years. Camillo, now in the service of Polixenes, begs the Bohemian king to allow him to return to Sicilia. Polixenes refuses and reports that his son, Prince Florizel, has fallen in love with a lowly shepherd girl, Perdita. He suggests to Camillo, to take his mind off thoughts of home, that they disguise themselves and attend the sheep-shearing feast where Florizel and Perdita will be betrothed. At the feast, hosted by the Old Shepherd, who has prospered thanks to the gold in the bundle, Autolycus picks the pocket of the Young Shepherd and, in various guises, entertains the guests with bawdy songs and trinkets. Disguised, Polixenes and Camillo watch as Florizel (under the guise of a shepherd named Doricles) and Perdita are betrothed. Then, tearing off the disguise, Polixenes angrily intervenes, threatening the Old Shepherd and Perdita with torture and death and ordering his son never to see the shepherd's daughter again. With the aid of Camillo, however, who longs to see his native land again, Florizel and Perdita set sail for Sicilia, using the clothes of Autolycus as a disguise. They are joined on their voyage by the Old Shepherd and his son, who are directed there by Autolycus.

In Sicilia, Leontes is still in mourning. Cleomenes and Dion plead with him to end his time of repentance because the kingdom needs an heir. Paulina, however, convinces the king to remain unmarried forever since no woman can match the greatness of his lost Hermione. Florizel and Perdita arrive, and they are greeted effusively by Leontes. Florizel pretends to be on a diplomatic mission from his father, but his cover is blown when Polixenes and Camillo also arrive in Sicilia. The meeting and reconciliation of the kings and princes happens, and it turns out that they learn that Old Shepherd raised Perdita. Leontes is reunited with his daughter, and he begs Polixenes for forgiveness. The Old Shepherd and Young Shepherd, now made gentlemen by the kings, meet Autolycus, who asks them for their forgiveness for his roguery. Leontes, Polixenes, Camillo, Florizel, and Perdita then go to Paulina's house in the country, where a statue of Hermione has been made. The sight of his wife's form makes Leontes upset, but then, to everyone's amazement, the statue moves. Hermione has been restored to life. As the play ends, Perdita and Florizel are engaged, and the whole company celebrates the miracle. Despite this happy ending, the unjust death of young prince Mamillius stays in everyone's mind, along with all the years wasted in separation.

In this play, the lead character, Leontes, suffers paranoia and hallucinations. He is similar to Othello, who was also paranoid about his wife having sex with someone else. Dr. Adler would point out that Leontes is struggling in masculine protest. Leontes also dominates the other men in the play. At the beginning, it is Polixenes who is his guest, then other men, like Camillo. He suffers for all this until the twists and turns of the play return his daughter and her new husband to him.

Ages of the Moon (2009) by Sam Shepard could be another play of male inadequacy and domination.

Two men, Byron and Ames, sit on a battered porch on a hot night and talk about old times. Occasionally, they sip their bourbon and stare into the darkness. There is going to be an eclipse in the early hours that they hope to see.

The play lasts little more than an hour and feels as if it should be paired with another piece. It's sentimental and doesn't feel much like a Shepard play. There's a tinge of wry humor. The mysteries of male friendship are hinted at.

7

Reich's Ideas

Dr. Wilhelm Reich (1897–1957) was also a student of Freud. His contributions to psychiatry include the study of character structure, the study of the psychology of fascism, and studies of sexuality. In opposition to Freud, Reich argued that every neurosis is the result of the damming up of sexual energy. Freud had suggested that at first but later considered neurosis to be a product of mental conflicts.

In his consideration of neurosis, Reich saw the whole model of sexuality as negated, turned into anxiety, so that humans are no longer able to fear pleasure as they usually did. Because the release of energy now falls under the threat of punishment, people may avoid pleasure and try to reach satisfaction with help of the hunger model. In choosing satiety over pleasure, humans fall into a system of voluntary servitude with wide-reaching political and socioeconomic consequences. Reich developed these concepts in *The Mass Psychology of Fascism*.[1]

This whole dynamic is, for Reich, the cause of masochism, which, once again, is not primary, but results from the blocking of libidinal movement. It is this mechanism that explains the person's reluctance against mental healing in therapy. According to Reich, patients have internalized a mechanism that rejects pleasure, so any release of libidinal energy, any pleasure, feels inherently wrong. Being mentally healthy would mean not feeling any anxiety, but people have so internalized morality that such a condition feels wrong to us. It is "good" to feel anxious, even though it does not *feel* good. The patients feel that it is their anxiety that keeps them together, that makes sure that they don't fall prey to their "primitive urges." They fear healing itself; for Reich, here is the biggest problem for analysis: to undo pleasure anxiety and to allow the patients to feel true pleasure again.

There are a few possible outcomes of this sexual inhibition according to Reich. One is neurotic symptoms and maladaptive character traits with body tensions. Also, Reich thought sexual energy is converted into anxiety and is

---

[1] Reich, Wilhelm, *The Mass Psychology of Fascism* (New York: Orgone Institute Press, 1933).

released in sadism or aggression. He believed societies can be aggressively sadistic like fascist Germany.

Reich pointed out that the hysterical character has the least number of defenses and the most lability of function. The hysteric is usually sexual and seductive in character.

Blanche DuBois in *A Streetcar Named Desire* by Tennessee Williams is a perfect example of a hysterical character in Reich's terms. She socializes by flirting with every man she meets. She's actually trying to maintain her dignity in this manner. Stanley Kowalski is Blanche's sister's husband. He sees right through Blanche. He must be sexually frustrated as well because he calls her bluff and ends up raping Blanche. This destroys all her limited defenses, so she must be taken to a mental hospital. Some say that this character was inspired by Williams's own mother.

Tennessee Williams (1911–1983) was born in Mississippi. He had diphtheria as a child and was not as strong as his father wanted him to be. In fact, Tennessee was quite weak and effeminate. His mother focused too much attention on him as a result. Rose, his sister, had schizophrenia, and since her behavior was so erratic and it was 1943, the doctors gave her a lobotomy. Williams took care of her the best he could and visited her when she was institutionalized. She is thought to be the model for Laura Wingfield in *The Glass Menagerie,* whereas Amanda Wingfield in the same play represents his mother.

In Neil LaBute's (1963–) play *Fat Pig*, the sadistic impulses of the playwright are let loose. A man falls in love with an overweight woman, and he is mocked by his fellow office workers. Because of the pressure of these colleagues, he breaks up with her. Throughout the play, we hear constant sadistic insults against the overweight character. Many of Neil LaBute's plays are similar to this one. Sadistic people insult a disabled or a "different" woman of some sort.

In the Company of Men by LaBute, two male employees of a big company are angry at women in general, so they try to find an insecure woman whom they will romance simultaneously and then leave her flat. Chad and Howard, the two men, choose Christine, a deaf coworker. Their schemes go astray in various ways, and Chad eventually breaks the news to her. He cruelly taunts her. There is a lot of sadism and aggression in these plays, probably because the characters are sexually frustrated, as Reich would explain it. LaBute is known in this way for breaking social graces and barriers. He is famous for being nasty, brutish, and uncouth in his works.

The play *In the Next Room*, or the *Vibrator* play, by Sarah Ruhl takes place in a seemingly perfect Victorian home with a proper gentleman and scientist Dr. Givings, who has invented a new device for treating women with hysteria. It's a vibrator. Of course, the women are dying to be treated by Dr. Givings because he brings them all to orgasm. Givings's own wife wonders what's going on when she hears all the commotion in the next room. Dr. Givings is cold and ungiving to Mrs. Givings. Dr. Reich would enjoy analyzing this play with all the pent-up sexual energy being released with the vibrator and the male hysteric, Dr. Givings.

Topdog/Underdog (2001) by Suzan-Lori Parks depicts two African American brothers dealing with racism, their work, women, and their childhoods. The brothers, Lincoln and Booth, were deserted when they were teens. Their parents left them $500 each, their inheritance. Lincoln works in whiteface as an Abraham Lincoln impersonator. In the past, they played three-card Monte or shoplifted to earn an illegal living. At the end, the brothers fight over their inheritance (Booth has kept his in a stocking). Booth shoots Lincoln for attempting to steal his money.

Dr. Reich would say that the brothers represent two sides of an unconscious conflict within the self. In gestalt therapy, a dialogue is encouraged between the top dog, the bullying, demanding, authoritarian side and the underdog, a dependent, compliant, but passively manipulative side. The dialogue is supposed to bring the two sides together and the patient takes responsibility. In Ms. Parks play, neither brother takes responsibility or realizes anything of importance, but their dialogue examines their relationship and how impossible life is for both of them.

Dr. Reich was an interesting character because of his theories about orgone (life force energy) and his development of the orgone box. He believed that constrictions of this life force caused cancer and other diseases, so he created a box that people could sit in to increase their orgone. The scientific community dismissed him as a crank, a pseudoscientist. He even persuaded Albert Einstein to talk to him for a few hours. He kept bothering Einstein after the initial meeting, but Einstein wouldn't answer him. The Federal Drug Administration obtained a federal injunction barring interstate distribution of orgone materials. Reich's therapists diagnosed him with "incipient psychosis," and one psychiatrist thought he had bipolar disorder. Nevertheless, Reich's theories of character structure and the psychology of fascism are still relevant to psychiatry.

Dr. Reich also had sex and relationships with several of his patients, a situation strictly forbidden in the fields of psychiatry and psychology. We consider our patients too vulnerable when they are under our care to be able to make a decision of whether to have sex or not with their therapists. Such intimacy is considered a major violation of boundaries and professional standards.

Many movies have depicted psychiatrists or psychologists seducing their patients. As one example, Sabina Spielrein in *A Dangerous Method* is seduced by her therapist, Carl Jung.

My play, *Under the Dragon* (2003), involves a psychiatrist, Dr. Greene, who falls in love with her patient, Peter, and then goes off to a hotel with him. At first, I didn't want to use this plot, but eventually I did after receiving a lot of feedback from my mentor and other students in a playwriting class I was taking. Fortunately, in the play I managed to conclude that the psychiatrist herself was a bipolar patient, and that she was in a manic phase, merely imagining the affair. She even thought her patient had jumped out the window of the hotel because she felt so guilty about thinking they had engaged in an affair. Her husband, a logical attorney, figures everything out and brings her the medications that help return her to reality.

Under the Dragon was one of my first plays. We first presented it in New York City at the Neighborhood Playhouse in 2002 and then had a reading of it at the United Nations theater in 2003.

Speed the Plow is a 1988 play by David Mamet. It's supposed to be a satirical dissection of the American movie business. Mamet did it better in his films.

The play begins in Bobby Gould's office. He is the new head of a big Hollywood film studio. His associate, Charlie Fox, brings him the great news that one of their movie stars, Doug Brown, wants to make a movie with them. The script was sent to him a while ago, and he could have gone to any studio. Gould's secretary (Madonna when I saw it) is sent out for coffee. The two men talk about her as if she's ripe for seduction. Fox bets $500 if Gould could seduce her. They are definitely crossing sexual boundaries here by treating her in this manner. In act 2, Karen goes to Gould's apartment to give him a review of a book they are considering to make into a movie. Instead of him seducing her, she seduces him, trying to convince him to make a movie from the novel. In act 3, Fox is back in Gould's office. Gould surprises him by telling Fox to forget about the script; he wants to make a movie from the book. When Karen arrives, Fox finds out that she only seduced Gould to influence him about the book. Her ambitious motives are revealed, and Fox forces her to leave. He then pitches the script to Gould again.

William Makepeace Thackeray wrote: "Which is the most reasonable, and does his duty best: he who stands aloof from the struggle of life, calmly contemplating it, or he who descends to the ground, and takes his part in the contest?"[2] The character of Bobby Gould finds himself on both sides of this dilemma, and at times in the play he "stands aloof," and at other times he "takes part" in life's contest, with its moral strictures.

The night I saw *Slave Play* (2018) by Jeremy O. Harris, the theater was packed. Everyone wanted to see this spectacle about interracial sex. The play is supposedly about three interracial couples undergoing "antebellum sexual performance therapy." The Black people no longer feel sexually attracted to their white partners. In act 1, Kaneisha, a Black slave, is twerking to a song when Jim, a white slave owner, comes in with a whip. Kaneisha calls him "Master," which Jim doesn't like. He berates her for the dirty room and commands her to eat a cantaloupe he throws on the floor. She eats it and dances, which arouses Jim. She wants to be called a "nasty, lazy negress." Jim performs cunnilingus on her instead. Next we're in the bedroom of Madame McGregor, the wife of Master McGregor, who wants her mulatto servant Phillip to play the fiddle. He plays music by Beethoven, which Madame McGregor doesn't like. She wants "Negro" music, so he plays "Pony" by Ginuwine. She dances, and then comes on to Phillip, and eventually sticks a dildo in his anus. Finally, in the barn, Gary, a Black slave, bosses around Dustin, a white indentured servant. Gary kicks Dustin down. They fight and then have sex. Gary makes Dustin lick his boots, which brings Gary to orgasm. After this, Patricia and Teá (therapists) arrive in modern outfits. They tell the three couples to meet back in the main house. The couples have each been in a role-playing exercise. In act 2, everyone in the cast tries to have a group therapy session to process what just happened, but it is the most inauthentic group session I've ever seen. Patricia and Teá speak academic jargon that is not even accurate. The couples talk about their fantasies and sexual inadequacies. The therapists say they are treating anhedonia, a psychological condition characterized by the inability to experience feelings of pleasure. The specific form of anhedonia featured in this play is purportedly caused by racial trauma passed down through history, causing Blacks to be unable

[2] Thackeray, William Makepeace, *Pendennis* (London, UK: Victorian Press, 1850).

to enjoy sex with whites due to "racialized inhibiting disorder" (not a real syndrome). The therapists in the play say people have anxiety, obsessive-compulsive disorder and musical obsession as a result. In act 3, Kaneisha declares that Jim never listens to her. She reviews their history and tells Jim she finds his whiteness frightening and that he is privileged. Jim calls her a "negress" and starts raping her until she calls out a "safeword" that they used in act 1. They wind up crying and laughing together, which seemed totally inappropriate.

Critics have either loved or hated this play. I thought it was ridiculous most of the time. The phony therapies, which were intended to transform all the weird sex into something palatable, took me out of the story completely. The playwright was trying to titillate the audience with all these sexual scenes to interest them and capture their attention instead of exploring these valid issues: Do Black and white people have trouble having sex with each other? Is the trauma of slavery passed down through the generations, causing sexual inhibitions or acting out? Would sex scenarios such as these help people overcome traumas and inhibitions?

Salome (1891) by Oscar Wilde was originally written in French. An English translation was done three years later, but the English banned the play because there were biblical characters.

Jokanaan (John the Baptist, Iokanaan in the original French text) is in jail because of his negative comments about Herodias, Herod's second wife. A young captain of the guard sees the beautiful princess Salome, Herod's stepdaughter, and longs for her, even though he is warned not to look at her because something terrible may happen. Salome is fascinated by Jokanaan's voice, and she persuades the captain to open the prison so that Jokanaan can get out. When he does, he denounces Herodias and her husband. Salome is frightened of him, but then she wants to touch his hair, his skin, and his lips. When she tells him she is Herodias's daughter, he calls her a "daughter of Sodom" and tells her to keep away. All Salome's attempts to attract him fail. He returns to his prison. The young captain of the guard, unable to bear Salome's desire for another man, fatally stabs himself.

Herod appears from the palace, looking for Salome. He slips in the captain's blood and panics. Herodias dismisses his fears and asks him to go back inside with her. Herod wants to seduce Salome, who rejects him. From his jail cell, Jokanaan resumes his criticism of Herodias. She demands that Herod hand the prophet over to the Jews. Herod refuses. He thinks that Jokanaan is a holy man. His words trigger an argument among the Jews about the true nature of God, and two Nazarenes talk about the miracles of Jesus. As Jokanaan continues to accuse her, Herodias demands that he be silenced.

Herod asks Salome to dance for him. She refuses, but when he promises to give her anything she wants, she agrees. Ignoring her mother's pleas, Salome performs the dance of the seven veils. Herod loves the dance and asks what reward Salome would like. She asks for the head of Jokanaan on a silver platter. Horrified, Herod refuses, while Herodias rejoices at Salome's choice. Herod offers other rewards, but Salome insists and reminds Herod of his promise. He finally yields. The executioner does the deed. When his head is brought to her, she passionately addresses Jokanaan as if he were still alive and finally kisses him.

Freudians would, of course, consider John the Baptist's beheading to be a symbol of castration. In Freudian psychoanalytic theory, castration is the whole combination of the child's unconscious feelings and fantasies associated with being deprived of the phallus, which in boys means the loss of the penis. Freud believed boys feared that their fathers would cut their penises off because they coveted their mothers in the oedipal stage (around three years old). In girls the Freudian belief was that the penis had already been removed. Modern psychoanalytical theory has moved on from assigning women castration complexes, but many old-fashioned analysts still adhere to the theory of castration anxiety in men.

In my play, *Lila's Penis*, the main character, Lila, who is a patient of the only other character, Dr. Sugar, is explaining to her psychiatrist that she has grown a penis. Dr. Sugar tries to reason with her to no avail because her patient is psychotic. At the end Lila tries to seduce Dr. Sugar with her new penis.

Lila's Penis

©2022 by Carol W. Berman

Setting: The present. A psychiatrist's office in which two chairs face each other. The patient, Lila, is an attractive young woman in her early twenties. The doctor, Dr. Sugar, is a relaxed woman in her fifties.

Lila

Why didn't anyone tell me that I could grow a penis? I mean how would you like to wake up one day and see a penis growing on you? What am I supposed to think? That I'm a hermaphrodite! I have enough bad stuff happening to me.

Dr. Sugar

Wait a second. A penis? Did you check it out with your doctor?

Lila

I don't need a doctor to tell me I have a penis. I've seen enough of them. Thank you.

Dr. Sugar

What does that mean to you—to think that you grew a penis?

Lila

I don't think I grew one. I grew one.

Dr. Sugar

How about going to your gynecologist and checking it out?

Lila

My mother showed me what she has to prove that I don't have a penis.

Dr. Sugar

What? Your mother did what?

Lila

My mother's weird. Like I've been telling you. She showed me her stuff.

Dr. Sugar

Of course, it's not appropriate. She should have just taken you to a doctor.

Lila

Well, at least guys won't be so eager to have sex with me.

Dr. Sugar

Are they so eager now?

Lila

What? Do I look ugly to you or something? A lot of guys hit on me all the time.

Dr. Sugar

So how do you respond?

Lila

It depends on the guy. Most of them I reject, but there have been a few that I went with.

Dr. Sugar

I thought you told me that you haven't been with a guy since high school.

Lila

I thought you wanted to hear that. I think my mother likes to hear that.

Dr. Sugar

I remind you of your mother?

Lila

Not really. You make a lot more sense.

Dr. Sugar

I'm glad you feel that I do.

Lila

But it's not helpful to try to talk me out of the fact that I grew a penis.

Dr. Sugar

Women don't just grow a penis out of nowhere. The logical thing would be to check with a gynecologist. It's probably a cyst or something like that.

Lila

You enjoy explaining things away. Maybe one day you wake up and you suddenly have a penis or one day you wake up and you've been turned into a cockroach.

Dr. Sugar

If you're talking about Kafka, the cockroach was a metaphor.

Lila

My penis isn't a metaphor. It's real.

Dr. Sugar

My job is to try to connect you to reality, Lila.

Lila

Why is reality so wonderful? It sucks if you ask me.

Dr. Sugar

In what way? What's bothering you?

Lila

I just told you. The new penis is disturbing me. Do I use the men's room or the ladies' room? Will other women shun me in the locker room? I can't go into the men's locker room because I still have breasts. I wonder if they'll shrink? I hope not.

[*She holds her hands under her breasts.*]

Dr. Sugar

You're asking important reality questions, which is a step in the right direction. What do hermaphrodites do? I think they usually choose one sex or another and go with that.

Lila

I'd rather be a woman. That's why this penis is disturbing.

Dr. Sugar

What do you like about being a woman?

Lila

Sex is much more relaxing as a woman. It seems like a big strain to be a man and worry about your penis standing up at the right time. I don't have to prove myself as a woman, although maybe I will now that I grew a penis. Maybe it's a punishment.

Dr. Sugar

Punishment for what?

Lila

I was doing it with guys.

Dr. Sugar

That's perfectly normal.

                              Lila

It's always "normal" or "real" with you, Dr. Sugar. That gets boring.

                            Dr. Sugar

Boring! We're not here to entertain each other. You're in treatment with me to
get into the real world.

                              Lila

I didn't know I was in treatment for that. I thought you were here to help me
feel better.

                            Dr. Sugar

You will feel better when you concentrate on reality.

                              Lila

I guess you can help me feel less upset that I grew a penis.
Maybe it's not lack of reality or a punishment.

                            Dr. Sugar

What do you think it is?

                              Lila

A gift?

                            Dr. Sugar

A gift?

                              Lila

Dr. Sugar, I think you should check it.

                            Dr. Sugar

That would be as bad as your mother looking at it. It's not appropriate. Call up
your gynecologist and ask to see her as soon as possible.

                              Lila

It's responding to you.

Dr. Sugar

What do you mean?

Lila

It's coming to life. I mean . . . it's, it's alive. This is what it must be like to be a man.

[*She gets out of her seat and starts coming toward the doctor.*]

Dr. Sugar

Take it easy, Lila. Please sit down.

BLACKOUT

8

Klein's Positions

Melanie Klein (1882–1960) was a psychoanalyst primarily responsible for object relations theory. She suffered from postpartum depression and did psychoanalysis in Vienna with Andor Ferenzi, who encouraged her to study psychoanalysis. She started the work by observing her own children. Klein developed "play technique," which was equivalent to free association in adults. Klein was trying to uncover the unconscious in children. Her marriage failed in 1921, and she moved to Berlin, where she joined the Berlin Psychoanalytical Society. There she continued her studies with Karl Abraham. She was a divorced woman who didn't even have a bachelor's degree, so her ideas were not well received in Berlin. Many of her theories conflicted with Freud's theories of development.

Anna Freud, Sigmund's daughter, was presenting her ideas around the same time. The two women became rivals. Amid these controversies, the British Psychoanalytical Society split into three divisions: (1) Kleinian; (2) Freudian; and (3) Independent. Anna Freud used an ego psychology approach. She published her famous monograph of defenses, *The Ego and the Mechanisms of Defense*, International Universities Press, Inc. Revised edition 1979, Madison, CT. In the early stages of childhood, defenses are developed as a result of the ego's struggles to mediate between the id and reality. She considered projection, denial, and distortion to be narcissistic defenses, while acting out, blocking, hypochondria, introjection, passive-aggressiveness, regression, schizoid fantasy, and somatization are immature defenses. Neurotic defenses would be controlling, displacement, dissociation, externalization, inhibition, intellectualization, isolation, rationalization, reaction formation, repression, and sexualization. Mature defenses consist of altruism, anticipation, asceticism, humor, sublimation, and suppression.

Klein's object relations theory is a variation of psychoanalytic theory. It places less emphasis on biological-based drives and more importance on interpersonal relationships. In object relations theory, objects are usually persons, parts of persons (e.g., the mother's breast), or symbols of one of these. The primary object is the mother. The child's relation to an object (e.g., the mother's breast) serves as the prototype for future interpersonal relationships. Objects can be both external (a physical person or body part) and internal, comprising emotional images and representations of an external object (e.g., good breast vs. bad breast).

The conceptualization of internal objects is linked to Klein's theory of unconscious fantasy and development from the paranoid-schizoid position to the depressive position.

Nicholas Wright (1940–) wrote a play called *Mrs. Klein*, which is set in London in 1934. The play begins with Melanie Klein attending the funeral of her son, Hans. Then the conflict between Melanie Klein and her daughter, Melitta, encompasses most of the play. Melitta accuses her mother, Mrs. Klein, of destroying Hans and propelling him toward suicide. Mrs. Klein is seen in a negative light by Melitta because she analyzed her two children. Melitta says her mother is totally bad and that she and her brother became emotional cripples from the analysis. In this play, Melitta (an analyst herself) views her mother as all bad. Melanie Klein thought that the child must split impulses and objects into all good and all bad to build an internal world. If an adult becomes stuck in the all good and all bad dynamic, then psychiatrists usually label the person with borderline personality disorder (BPD).

The infant cannot perceive the mother at all but is only aware of her breasts. The infant then splits the world into the "good breast" and the "bad breast." The good breast provides nourishment to the child, and the bad breast withholds that nourishment. (Klein's assumption was that the child is breastfed, but this also applies to a bottle that is given or withheld.) This division into good and bad is called splitting. Klein described two major constellations: the paranoid-schizoid position and the depressive position. In the first one, the paranoid-schizoid position, there is a predominance of splitting and part object relationships and a basic fear of survival of the ego or self. In the second one, which evolves later, the depressive position appears, in which the child sees that the good and bad are really one.

Melanie Klein believed that at about six months of age splitting begins to decline. It is then that a child becomes aware that the good and bad external objects are really one. Then the infant can acknowledge his own aggression toward a good object or recognize good aspects of a bad object he's attacking. She thought that the basic fear about good inner and external objects surviving must be preserved even at the expense of the ego. Internal bad objects are no longer projected and become the superego, which can then attack the ego with guilt.

Birthday Candles (2022) by Noah Haidle explores the life of a character called Ernestine from eighteen to one hundred years old. Each passing year or sometimes decade is introduced with a bell. Ernestine is always in the kitchen (the only set) trying to make a birthday cake. Various characters (i.e., her mother, husband, children, grandchildren, etc.) pass through her life. At first, I considered the play mawkishly sentimental and too stereotypical, but I soon realized Haidle was employing all these devices and characters to make a point about the brevity of existence and the repetition of life patterns throughout the years. How life passes in a flash, how each generation experiences the same traumas of birth, relationships, and death. Ernestine is the perfect mother, the good breast as Klein would describe her. She was always loving, patient, and thankful. The only time she was the bad breast was when her husband, Matt, strayed from the marriage. Even then she was silent and unrealistically stoic. She even nurses him when he gets dementia. The play is a parable based on Thornton Wilder's *The Long Christmas Dinner* (1931), in which we witness ninety years and are accelerated through ninety Christmas dinners in the Bayard home. We see changes in customs and manners during this time and the growth of the Bayard family, all typical of American life. The ending of *Birthday Candles* is especially poignant when we find Ernestine (at one hundred) in the kitchen as usual, trying to prepare her birthday cake, but we soon discover that she has escaped from a nursing home to return to her house, which now harbors a young couple. She finally dies and sees her mother and the rest of the family.

We often talk about narcissism and narcissistic personality disorder (NPD). Otto Kernberg, a famous psychoanalyst and professor of psychiatry, followed the work of Melanie Klein and helped to develop many theories about narcissism. He stated there were three types of narcissism: (1) normal adult narcissism (which we all have to a lesser or greater extent); (2) normal infantile narcissism; and (3) pathological narcissism. He felt that the third (pathological narcissism) is a libidinal investment in a pathological structure of the self. Again, he divided this third, malignant, condition into thirds: (1) regression to the regulation of the infantile self-esteem; (2) narcissistic choice of object; and (3) NPD (the most severe). In the unconscious, the self is a structure made up of many self-representations, according to object relations theories. A realistic self or ego can integrate the good and bad self-images, but one with an NPD is stuck. In normal adult narcissism, the healthiest situation, the person has introjected whole representations of objects and has them stabilized into a solid moral system. The superego, ego, and id all work well together. In normal infantile narcissism, self-esteem is regulated through an infantile set of values, demands, and prohibitions. However, in pathological narcissism, there is regression to infantile self-esteem, in which the ego is dominated by infantile pursuits. When there is a narcissistic object of choice, the unconscious projects itself onto someone and then identifies with him or her.

The worst-case scenario is the NPD, in which the ego is defending against early self and objects that are held in the unconscious with aggression and libidinal destructive forces. Kernberg remained faithful to Freud and Klein. Unlike his colleague Kohut, Kernberg thought narcissistic and borderline personalities had similar defenses of splitting and projective identification. Kohut saw BPD as different from NPD. He thought BPD was impossible to treat, whereas Kernberg believed they were both treatable.

Shakespeare wrote *Henry VIII* in 1613 about the real king, who had been considered a perfect example of a narcissist since he reigned. The duke of Buckingham and other lords discuss the meeting of King Henry and the French king in the prologue of the play. Then, Buckingham is unexpectedly arrested for treason. At court, King Henry makes decisions about woolen trade with his wife, Queen Katharine. She then pleads in behalf of Buckingham, which Henry won't hear, and he orders the duke's trial. Cardinal Wolsey, who betrayed the duke, holds a feast in his palace; the king and his friends arrive disguised as shepherds. Wolsey recognizes him. Henry dances with Anne Boleyn. In the next act, Buckingham is condemned to be executed by false witnesses. The court gossip spreads that Wolsey has too much power and is trying to break up Henry and Katharine. Wolsey, Henry, and some other religious figures discuss if Henry's marriage is valid and the possibility of divorce.

Queen Katharine wants to obtain advisors from Spain, her native country, when she must face a divorce trial. Wolsey refuses to allow this, and she leaves accusing the cardinal of stirring up Henry. Wolsey goes after her when she's with her ladies and forces her to submit to the divorce. Henry secretly marries Anne Boleyn, who was a lady to the queen. Then Henry learns that Wolsey secretly wrote to the pope to oppose the divorce. Henry forces Wolsey to give up his role as lord chancellor. Queen Anne is crowned. She gives birth to Elizabeth, who is baptized and prophesied to become a great queen.

King Henry VIII went on to have four other wives and to rid himself of them when and as he saw fit. In the Shakespeare play, he has no consideration for Queen Katharine and hardly any for Anne Boleyn. As an NPD, he has a grandiose sense of himself; he's preoccupied with fantasies of unlimited power and ideal love; he believes he's special (he is, of course), and he requires excessive admiration and allegiance. One could say he was a king, so none of this applies, but being a king's (Henry VII) son also, he probably didn't have a lot of nurturing, so Kernberg's criteria of NPD apply.

King Henry demonstrates the primitive defense mechanism of splitting. Such a mechanism is normal in children before six months of age and in certain personality disorders, such as NPD and BPD. Good and bad objects are kept apart, or split. Good objects are introjected, while bad objects are projected. Henry projects bad onto his old queen, Katharine, and good onto his new queen, Anne. He did this several times whenever he was ready to discard the old queen and get a new one.

Who's Afraid of Virginia Woolf? is a play by Edward Albee (1928–2016), first staged in 1962. It examines the complexities of the marriage of a middle-aged couple, Martha and George. Late one evening, after a university faculty party, they receive an unwitting younger couple, Nick and Honey, as guests and draw them into their bitter and frustrated relationship.

The play is in three acts, normally taking a little less than three hours to perform. The title is a pun on the song "Who's Afraid of the Big Bad Wolf?" Albee substitutes the famous author for the bad wolf. Martha and George sing this song throughout the play while they engage in horrible emotional games. He is a professor of history, and she is the daughter of the president of the college where George teaches. When Nick and Honey arrive, Martha and George insult each other as everyone gets drunk. Martha is aggressive, while George is passive-aggressive. The evening continues with George breaking a bottle, Honey throwing up, and everyone disturbed. George and Nick talk about children and birth and death in act 2. Finally, George starts to insult his guests, calling Honey "the Mousie." Martha comes on to Nick and goes upstairs to bed with him. In act 3, George and Martha talk about their nonexistent son. George and Martha have played this game about their son since they learned they were infertile. George "killed" him in a story he made up because Martha was not supposed to mention the son to anyone else. Nick and Honey finally leave, horrified at this crazy couple's antics. Martha wants to make up another imaginary child, but George forbids it. He says it's time they ended the game.

George and Martha are each other's bad objects, so they constantly torture each other as they project one horrible thing after another onto each other. They finally engage Nick and Honey in their primitive projections. Alcohol fuels their fury. The innocent young couple have never seen anything like George and Martha, although their psyches are not particularly coherent either.

George Bernard Shaw (1856–1950) wrote more than sixty plays and was awarded the Nobel Prize in Literature in 1925. *Arms and the Man* (1894) was his first public success. The title comes from the opening of Virgil's Aeneid: "Of arms and the man I sing." It's 1885 in the play, during the Serbo-Bulgarian War. Raina Petkoff is a young Bulgarian woman engaged to Serguis Saranoff, a hero of the war. She idolizes him. Captain Bluntschli climbs in through Raina's window one night and tells her to be quiet or he'll shoot her. Russian and Bulgarian troops burst into her house to search for the captain, but Raina hides him. Bluntschli is practical and cynical about war, which shocks Raina, who's idealistic about it. She and her mother sneak him out of the house wearing Raina's father's coat when the troops leave. Bulgarians and Serbs sign a peace treaty, so Raina's father, Major Paul Petkoff, and Serguis return home. Serguis strikes Raina as a fool and boring, but she doesn't let him know she feels like this. Serguis feels the same way about her. He flirts with the servant girl, Louka, who is engaged to Nicola, another servant. Bluntschli returns to give Raina her father's coat that he'd borrowed. Raina's father and boyfriend, Serguis, know Bluntschli, who stays for lunch. Raina had left him a note saying he's a chocolate cream soldier. Raina and Bluntschli like each other, and he proposes to her when he learns she's 23. He's 34 and thought she was younger. His father died and left him several luxury hotels in Switzerland, where he's from originally and where he's returning. Serguis proposes to Louka to everyone's amazement. Raina wanted Bluntschli when he was her poor "chocolate cream soldier," and she hesitates to say yes to him because he's become a rich businessman. Bluntschli says he's the same person, and Raina finally agrees to marry him.

This play is a light comedy with a lot of Shaw's wit, but he makes many important points: (1) That war is not romantic, but it's horrible; (2) class distinctions, which were so important at his time, are ridiculous; (3) love is fickle and can change in a minute.

We don't delve deeply into any of the characters in Shaw's plays, but we don't need to. We understand who everyone is quickly and what they want. The soldiers (Raina's father; boyfriend, Serguis; and Bluntschli) all want to lead conventional lives after their traumatic experiences in the war. They may have post-traumatic stress disorder, so a regular home life for each of them would be soothing and healing. Raina is an idealistic dreamer who has been protected by her upper-class upbringing. She gets an abrupt awakening by Bluntschli when he climbs through her window and demands to be protected. This awakening allows her to see her fiancé, Serguis, clearly and to disconnect from him. He was the good object, but when she really sees him, he becomes the bad object; then, she can see that he's not the man for her after all. Serguis, in turn, sees her as a spoiled rich girl (the bad object) after his war experiences, so he turns to the maid, Louka, who is down-to-earth and the good object.

Shaw was a socialist, so he loved to show us characters disgusted with the upper-class life (e.g., *Pygmalion*, 1913). In this play, Professor Higgins teaches Eliza, a flower girl, to speak properly. Higgins says he can pass Eliza off as a duchess when he teaches her proper English. Colonel Pickering, a colleague from India, makes a bet with him and says he'll pay for Eliza's lessons if Higgins succeeds. Eliza becomes objectified by both of them. Higgins wins the bet, and they ignore Eliza and her feelings about the whole thing. She wonders what she will do with her life now, and she walks out on Higgins and Pickering. Eliza wins at the end and marries Freddy Eynsford-Hill, a gentleman.

All My Sons (1947) by Arthur Miller was his work questioning the "American dream," an idealization of our country and its ideals or as Klein would say the good breast.

The play starts in the middle of the action. In August 1946, Joe Keller, a self-made businessman, and his wife Kate are visited by a neighbor, Frank. At Kate's request, Frank is trying to figure out the horoscope of the Keller's missing son Larry, who disappeared three years earlier while serving in the military during World War II. There has been a storm, and the tree planted in Larry's honor has blown down during the month of his birth, making it seem that Larry is still alive. While Kate still believes Larry is coming back, the Keller's other son, Chris, doesn't believe it. Furthermore, Chris wishes to propose to Ann Deever, who was Larry's girlfriend at the time he went missing and who has been corresponding with Chris for two years. Joe and Kate react to this news with shock but are interrupted by Bert, the boy next door. He tattles to Joe and wants to see the "jail." In a game, Bert brings up the word "jail," making Kate react sharply. When Ann arrives, it is revealed that her father, Steve Deever, is in prison for selling cracked cylinder heads to the Air Force, causing the deaths of twenty-one pilots. Joe was his partner but was exonerated of the crime. Ann admits that neither she nor her brother keep in touch with their father anymore and wonders aloud whether a faulty engine was responsible for Larry's death. After a heated argument, Chris breaks in and later proposes to Ann, who accepts. Chris also reveals that while serving in the army he lost all his men and is experiencing survivor's guilt. Meanwhile, Joe receives a phone call from George, Ann's brother, who is coming there to settle something.

In act 2, Chris and Ann have become engaged, but Chris avoids telling his mother. Their next-door neighbor Sue emerges, revealing that everyone on the block thinks Joe is equally guilty of the crime of supplying faulty aircraft engines. Shortly afterward, George Deever arrives and reveals that he has just visited the prison to see his father, Steve. The latter has confirmed that Joe told him by phone to paint over the cracked cylinder heads and to send them out, and he later gave a false promise to Steve that he would account for the shipment on the day of arrest. George insists his sister, Ann, cannot marry Chris Keller, son of the man who destroyed the Deevers. Meanwhile, Frank reveals his horoscope, implying that Larry is alive, which is just what Kate wants to hear. Joe maintains that on the fateful day of dispatch, the flu laid him up, but Kate says that Joe has not been sick in fifteen years. Despite George's protests, Ann sends him away.

When Kate claims to Chris (who is still intent on marrying Ann) that moving on from Larry will be forsaking Joe as a murderer, Chris concludes that George was right. Joe, out of excuses, explains that he sent out the cracked cylinder heads to avoid closure of the business, intending to no- tify the base later that they needed repairs. However, when the fleet crashed and made headlines, he lied to Steve and abandoned him at the factory to be arrested. Chris cannot accept this explanation and exclaims in despair that he is torn about what to do about his father now.

In act 3, Chris has left home. Reluctantly accepting the accusations against her husband, Kate says that, should Chris return, Joe must express willing- ness to go to prison in the hope that Chris will relent. As he only sought to make money at the insistence of his family, Joe is adamant that their relation- ship is above the law. Soon after, Ann emerges and expresses her intention to leave with Chris regardless of Kate's disdain. When Kate angrily refuses again, Ann reveals to Kate a letter from Larry. She had not wanted to share it, but knows that Kate must face reality. Chris returns and is torn about whether to turn Joe in to the authorities, knowing it doesn't erase the death of his fellow soldiers or absolve the world of its natural merciless state.

When Joe returns and excuses his guilt on account of his life's accomplishments, his son says he saw him as the ideal father (the good breast). Finally, the letter, read by Chris, reveals that because of his father's guilt, Larry planned to commit suicide. With this final blow, Joe agrees to turn himself in. When Joe goes inside to get his coat, he kills himself with a gunshot off stage. At the end, when Chris expresses remorse in spite of his resolve, Kate tells him not to blame himself and to move on with his life.

Both sons idealized their father, Joe, and believed in the American dream, but the truth comes out that their father is less than ideal. He covered up faulty parts that were used and that killed soldiers as a result. Then he lies and lets his partner take the blame for the problem. His only solution is jail or suicide, and I was not surprised that he killed himself at the end. When idealization is broken in this way, people cannot live with themselves if they are in a primitive state in which they have not synthesized the good and bad breasts.

In Miller's plays, there are vital connections between the individual, the family, and society. These are prevalent in *Death of a Salesman* and *The Crucible*, as well as *All My Sons*. When those connections fail, there is no way out for individuals. I believe Miller was concerned with these relationships because at the time when he was a child and a teenager, Jewish families were attempting to blend into American society the best they could. His father was an immigrant who at first was successful in business, but then lost everything during the 1929 crash. Jews could not enter American society so easily in that time period, and there was extreme prejudice against them. When Hitler was fomenting his hatred in the 1930s, many Americans (including Charles Lindbergh) became pro-Nazi. Jewish families stuck together to help counteract the prejudice against them. Miller's plays show families trying to survive as society presses down on them. In *All My Sons*, the father wants to support his family, but he has been corrupted in his eagerness to prosper and produce parts. His fatal mistakes come to light, and he is destroyed as an ideal, as the good breast. His only choice is to destroy himself.

9

Personality Disorders

The many ego defenses elaborated by Anna Freud in the previous chapter show us how a person deals with stressful situations and how people defend against various threats to themselves. Character traits are related to the defense system but play a greater role in how a person functions.

Personality disorders are inflexible, lasting patterns of thinking, feeling, and behavior.[1] People with any of these personality disorders are stuck. They act against themselves or others, but they can't adapt to new situations and environments.

The old-fashioned categorizing of personality disorders does not help us with predicting clinical outcomes or in treatment planning. Researchers and clinicians are concerned that the diagnosis of a personality disorder has a negative connotation, and patients are treated poorly by doctors, hospitals, and insurance companies. There is also the problem of diagnostic reliability, co-occurrence, and inconsistent and arbitrary boundaries. Many say that there are inadequate scientific bases for the personality disorders. A good solution to the problem may be to look at various personality traits on a spectrum. Does the patient have a negative or positive affect? Is the person extroverted or introverted? Is the individual antagonistic or compliant, constrained or impulsive? There may be as many as eighteen different models for a dimensional proposal.

Many researchers are still arguing about how many factors are needed to represent differences in personality. Most people agree that the four dimensions of anxious-submissive, psychopathic, socially withdrawn, and compulsive are equivalent to neuroticism, disagreeableness, introversion/extraversion, psychoticism and conscientiousness. Factor analysis has identified passive, dependent, sociopathic, anankastic, and schizoid features. Any classification system needs to score severity of any of these factors.

Sadistic personality disorder appeared in the third edition of the *Diagnostic and Statistical Manual of Mental Disorders* (*DSM-IIIR*), but later

---

[1] Berman, Carol W., *Personality Disorders* (New York: Lippincott, Williams & Wilkins, 2009), p. 3.

versions of the diagnostic manual (fourth edition [*DSM-IV*], text revision of the fourth edition [*DSM-IV-TR*], and fifth edition [*DSM-5*]) did not include it. Psychiatrists did not want to have a category for sadistic personality disorder because of the controversy surrounding defining sexual disorders and possibly giving sadists a legal excuse. Basically, a sadistic person derives pleasure by making others suffer sexually, emotionally, or physically.

The Pillowman by Martin McDonagh is a good example of many characters using sadism. A fiction writer, Katurian, living in a police state, is interrogated about the horrible content of his short stories. They resemble a number of weird child murders in town. The cops, Ariel and Tupolski, torture Katurian, trying to get him to confess to these unsolved murders. Katurian tells the cops that he had a happy childhood with loving parents, but his brother was tortured nightly by his parents, and he heard it. Then Katurian and his brother are in a cell together. The writer tells his brother the story of *The Pillowman*, a man made of pillows who convinces children to kill themselves. The brother confesses to murdering the children in town because of the writer's stories. Katurian smothers his brother and then confesses to the murders.

When I saw the play on Broadway in 2005, I was cringing most of the time. There was no character I could relate to. Katurian, his brother, and the two cops are all sadistic, enjoying torturing each other.

In *Wit*, Margaret Edson shows us an English professor, Dr. Vivian Bearing, struck by ovarian cancer. She is undergoing experimental chemotherapy. Vivian's "wit" and knowledge of all the wonders of the English language do her no good as she struggles through her final hours in the hospital. Vivian recites John Donne's sonnet, "Death Be Not Proud." Vivian is the ultimate intellectual, rigid, obsessive-compulsive personality. She sees the same traits in the doctors around her. She has no family; her parents are deceased. She has no emergency contact. What she needs is kindness and care, and that's finally provided by Dr. Ashford, another woman professor of English literature and Vivian's former professor/mentor, who reads her a child's book and crawls into the hospital bed with Vivian to comfort her at the end.

People with an obsessive-compulsive personality disorder (OCDPD) are preoccupied by details, rules, order, and schedules. They are devoted to work to the exclusion of leisure and friends. Moreover, they are overconscientious and inflexible about ethics and values.[2] Vivian fits this description; so do

---

[2] Berman, *Personality Disorders*, p. 43.

most of the doctors she meets in the hospital. The play won the 1999 Pulitzer Prize for drama.

When I took my medical students to see the revival of *Wit* in 2012, I had a great opportunity to teach them about the OCD (obsessive-compulsive disorder) personality. Through this play, they were shown how a patient struggles to remain a human being in the hospital, stripped of all their usual defenses. Most important, I had a chance to teach them about the power of compassion and empathy in the treatment of patients. The willingness on the part of the medical team to extend their own vulnerable humanity to a patient is especially essential in end-of-life cases in which doctors have no weapons left to continue a fight.

In *Six Degrees of Separation* by John Guare, a young con man, Paul, insinuates himself into the life of Ouisa and Flan Kittredge, a wealthy New York couple. Paul says he's the son of Sidney Poitier. He claims he's been mugged, and all his money is gone. The Kittredges take him in and patch up his minor stab wound. Paul claims he's a friend of their children at Harvard. He's lying, and Ouisa and Flan only discover this when they catch Paul in bed with a hustler and then kick him out. He does another con with a naïve young couple, Rick and Elizabeth from Utah, seducing Rick and getting all their money. Elizabeth is enraged, and Rick commits suicide. Paul calls the Kittredges, and Ouisa responds to him but wants him to turn himself in to the police. Ouisa has a monologue at the end in which she says we are connected to everyone by only six other people—hence, the name of the play—but she wants to find the right six people.

Paul is a classic case of someone with an antisocial personality disorder.[3] He fails to conform to social norms of lawful behavior. He is deceitful, impulsive, irritable, and aggressive. He has a reckless disregard for the safety of himself or others. He's irresponsible and has no remorse about conning others. On top of everything, Paul is very intelligent, like a lot of con men.

Paul may also have borderline personality disorder (BPD). BPD is a chronic condition that may include mood instability, difficulty with interpersonal relationships, and high rates of self-injurious or suicidal behavior. BPD is characterized by pervasive instability in moods, interpersonal relationships, self-image, and behavior. This instability often disrupts family and work life, long-term planning, and an individual's sense of identity. People with BPD, originally thought to be at the "border" of psychosis and neurosis, suffer

---

[3] Berman, *Personality Disorders*, p. 17.

from difficulties with regulating their emotions. While less well known than schizophrenia or bipolar disorder, BPD affects two percent of adults. People with BPD exhibit high rates of self-injurious behavior, such as cutting, and elevated rates of attempted and completed suicide. Impairment from BPD and suicide risk are greatest in the young adult years and tend to decrease with age. BPD is more common in women than in men, with seventy-five percent of cases diagnosed among women.

People with BPD often need extensive mental health services and account for twenty percent of psychiatric hospitalizations. Yet, with help, the majority of people who suffer stabilize and lead productive lives.

The fact that Paul is Black, "the son of Sidney Poitier," may present problems in this era of Black Lives Matter. This is a clichéd trope of the Black con man working his way into white society, although when there were few opportunities for Blacks to advance in society, his behavior makes sense. The psychiatric definitions of personality disorders do not consider aspects like race, religion, or other identifying factors.

In *Othello* by Shakespeare (see Chapter 2), the main character exhibits paranoid personality disorder (PPD). People with PPD are always on guard, believing that others are constantly trying to demean, harm, or threaten them. These generally unfounded beliefs, as well as their habits of blame and distrust, might interfere with their ability to form close relationships. People with this disorder doubt the commitment, loyalty, or trustworthiness of others, believing others are using or deceiving them. They are reluctant to confide in others or reveal personal information due to a fear that the information will be used against them. They tend to be unforgiving and hold grudges and are hypersensitive and take criticism poorly. In addition, they can read hidden meanings in the innocent remarks or casual looks of others. Othello is a perfect example of a person with PPD, and all those around him suffer as a consequence. Othello could not see his role in problems or conflicts and believed he was always right. He was hostile, stubborn, and argumentative.

The exact cause of PPD is not known, but it likely involves a combination of biological and psychological factors. The fact that PPD is more common in people who have close relatives with schizophrenia suggests a genetic link between the two disorders. Early childhood experiences, including physical or emotional trauma, are also suspected to play a role in the development.

The *Hot L Baltimore* is a play by Lanford Wilson (1937–2011) that takes place in the lobby of the old, rundown Hotel Baltimore. The residents are faced with eviction because the building has been condemned. The play was written in 1973 and premiered at Circle in the Square Theater in New York City. Two prostitutes and various other characters struggle with the inevitable destruction of their home. The play depicts real people trying to survive in a decaying environment. Of course, we all have to face change and decay. Wilson's characters are down to earth and do the best they can. Some of them have personality disorders that do not help them in their struggles. I cannot say exactly which personality disorders they have since Mr. Wilson did not follow the *DSM-5* in his depictions of these characters, but like all people with rigid personality structures, they are handicapped to begin with.

Lanford Wilson received the Pulitzer Prize for drama in 1980. He wrote about junkies, prostitutes, and thieves, who often have personality disorders. In 1965, he wrote plays for Ellen Stewart's La MaMa Experimental Theatre Club. *Balm in Gilead* premiered there in 1965. I saw this amazing play in 1984, when the Circle Repertory Company and Steppenwolf Theatre Company put it on. It was an amazing production directed by John Malkovich. *Balm in Gilead* is set in Frank's café, a greasy spoon diner. Joe, a drug dealer, and Darlene, a naïve new arrival in the city, get together for sex, but then Joe rejects her. She's an easy target for various lowlifes in that area. I would say that Joe has a sociopathic personality disorder, while Darlene has more of a dependent personality disorder (DPD). They are both stuck, and at the end, all the characters are droning their lines from the first scene over and over in an endless, hopeless circle.

An individual with DPD has a neediness that is marked by an overreliance on others. His or her emotional and physical needs are dependent on the people to whom the person is closest. DPD is a pervasive and excessive need to be cared for that leads to submissive and clinging behavior as well as fears of separation. This pattern begins by early adulthood and is present in a variety of contexts. The dependent and submissive behaviors are designed to elicit care and arise from a self-perception of being unable to function adequately without the help of others.

Individuals with DPD have great difficulty making everyday decisions (e.g., what clothes to wear) without a lot of advice and reassurance from others. These individuals tend to be passive and allow other people (normally one other person) to take the initiative and assume responsibility for most major areas of their lives. Adults with this disorder typically depend on a parent, spouse, boyfriend, or girlfriend to decide where they should live, what kind of job they should have, and which people to befriend.

People with DPD seek support and approval and therefore cannot express opinions or disagreement, especially with those they are dependent on. They feel so unable to function alone that they will agree with things that they feel are wrong rather than risk losing the help of those to whom they look for guidance. Individuals with this disorder find it difficult to initiate projects or work independently.

They may go to extreme lengths to obtain nurturance and support from others, even to the point of volunteering for unpleasant tasks if such behavior will bring the care that they need. Individuals with this disorder feel uncomfortable or helpless when alone because of their exaggerated fears of being unable to care for themselves.

The condition is inflexible and maladaptive and can cause dysfunction and distress, as we see in Darlene's case in *Balm in Gilead*.

I Am My Own Wife (2003) by Doug Wright is a unique play about an East German transvestite called Charlotte von Mahlsdorf who lived under the Nazis and then the communists during her lifetime. She was born in 1928 as Lothar Berfelde, but grew up always thinking of herself as a female trapped in a man's body. Doug Wright actually traveled to where Charlotte lived in Mahlsdorf outside Berlin and interviewed her. He even obtained Stasi files on her and understood that she complied with the Stasi so that she could preserve her museum and lifestyle. To wit, she spied on her comrades. Mr. Wright wanted to just view her as a righteous artist, but he had to admit to her negative side as well. He composed his play from his interviews with Charlotte, but he appropriated a technique that director Moises Kaufman used in his play *The Laramie Project* and felt guilty for doing so. Wright used one actor to play all the parts. It made sense to him because Charlotte had to adopt all these guises to survive.

When I saw the play on Broadway in 2003, I was amazed that the actor Jefferson Mays was able to portray all these parts with just a change of voice, body stance, lighting, and good direction (by Moises Kaufman). He hardly changed costumes. The performance reminded me of patients with dissociative identity disorder (DID), previously known as multiple personality disorder (MPD), in which a patient maintains at least two distinct personality states.[4] There are usually memory gaps since the person has experienced neglect or trauma in childhood. Some patients have up to 100 different

---

[4] American Psychiatric Association, *Diagnostic and Statistical Manual of Mental Disorders* (5th ed.) (Washington, DC: American Psychiatric Association, 2013).

identities, although the actor in *I Am My Own Wife* only portrayed about thirty-five. There is even a psychiatrist in the play, Dr. Dieter Jorgensen, who says that Charlotte von Mahlsdorf suffers from autism because she "recounts her stories in a highly ritualized, cadenced way, less to communicate content than to provide a kind of rhythmic reassurance to the chaos in her psyche. This is true of autistic adults—repetition is a palliative. Her stories aren't lies, per se; they're self-medication."[5] I don't agree. There's nothing autistic about Charlotte in this play. In autism, a person has difficulties interacting socially, so they exhibit restricted and repetitive behaviors. Autism is a neurodevelopmental disorder usually seen in young children who don't meet the normal milestones of development, starting at six months. Charlotte, on the other hand, was able to not only run a museum and cabaret, but also fool both Nazi and Stasi agents—an extraordinary feat in itself, one that requires considerably advanced social skills.

Top Girls by Caryl Churchill (1982) seems to be a feminist play. There are only women in the cast, and a few are famous ones (i.e., Isabella Bird, Pope Joan, Patient Griselda, and Lady Nijo). Written at the time that Margaret Thatcher was prime minister, Ms. Churchill portrays her main character, Marlene, like Ms. Thatcher, a tough career woman who exploits other women, caring only about her own success. Marlene can be seen as having a narcissistic personality disorder.

The play opens with Marlene meeting Pope Joan, who was supposed to have ruled from 854 to 856 until she had a baby and was thereby discovered to have been a woman. They stoned her to death after that discovery. Isabella Bird, a world traveler, did not marry young because of her career. She abandoned her sister to advance herself. Lady Nijo, a thirteenth-century Japanese concubine, felt honored to sleep with the emperor at that time, but Marlene says it was rape and that the emperor considered her status as that of a prostitute. Patient Griselda, from Chaucer's *Canterbury Tales*, who was chosen to be the wife of the marquis, must always obey him. She is a poor peasant woman who, after several years of marriage, gives birth to a baby girl. When the baby is six weeks old, the marquis orders his wife to give the baby up, which she does. She also has to give up her baby son when he is two years old. After many more years, the marquis tells her to go home. Once home, she sees her children playing happily together and finally realizes that the marquis was testing her obedience.

[5] Wright, Doug, *I Am My Own Wife* (New York: Faber & Faber, 2004), p. 75.

The women discuss these men and their lives with them in act 1, scene 1. However, they hardly let each other speak and instead interrupt each other constantly. Are they all narcissists? Marlene is celebrating her promotion at the Top Girls Employment Agency. Then in the next scene, Marlene is back at her agency interviewing Jeanine, whom she likes for no reason except that Jeanine is the opposite of herself, an innocent woman content to just marry and have a baby. Scene 3, which is completely different from the first two scenes, features two young girls, Angie and Kit, discussing sex and sleeping around. Neither knows what she's talking about. In act 2, two women are gossiping when Marlene enters. We see Louise, who was only dedicated to work and has no family life. In the last scene, a year earlier, Marlene is with her sister, Joyce, and niece, Angie, sharing stories. The play ends with the audience understanding that Marlene gave Angie, who is really her daughter, to her sister Joyce, who lost her own unborn child from stress.

When I saw the play in 2007, I was thoroughly confused at the beginning because the women kept interrupting each other and telling such bizarre stories. I eventually caught on that Ms. Churchill was demonstrating how "top girls," or dominant women, struggle and compete throughout history. Was she saying that women become the patriarchy when they grasp for power and are ambitious? Or was she demonstrating how narcissistic women or men must be to survive in our world?

The Beauty Queen of Leenane (1996) by Martin McDonagh is about Maureen, a 40-year-old spinster, who lives in the Irish village of Leenane with her 70-year-old mother, Mag. Maureen is her mother's caregiver. While Maureen is out, Ray Dooley, a young man, invites both women to a farewell party for his visiting uncle. Ray writes the invitation down for Maureen because it seems that Mag doesn't get what he's saying. As soon as he leaves, Mag burns the note. Maureen returns and criticizes her mother for being so dependent on her. Maureen has a bad back and burnt hand, and she believes Mag can do more than she lets on. Maureen knows about the party from Ray, whom she passed on her way in, so she punishes Mag by forcing her to drink a horrible energy drink. Maureen is a virgin who has only kissed two men in her life. She attends the party in a new dress and then brings Ray's older brother, Pato, home with her. Pato, a construction worker, always thought of Maureen as "the beauty queen of Leenane." She has sex with him in her bedroom.

In the morning, Mag empties her bedpan into the kitchen sink, a daily habit that disgusts Maureen. Pato emerges from the bedroom and prepares breakfast for a shocked Mag. Maureen then comes out in her underwear and flaunts the fact that she slept with Pato. Mag is so mad that she accuses Maureen of having deliberately burnt her hand. She also tells Pato that she (Mag) is taking care of her daughter, not the other way around. Mag checked Maureen out of a mental hospital. Maureen admits that she truly did suffer a breakdown when she was in England, 15 years earlier. She claims Mag sometimes tells lies about the past, thinking Maureen can't tell the lies from the truth. Pato is sympathetic, telling her that his opinion of her is unchanged. He urges her to dress herself, which causes her to become insecure, and she starts to scream. Mag enters with documents to prove that Maureen was in the hospital, but Pato ignores her. He leaves, saying he will write to Maureen.

Pato does write from London, where he works, but he says that he is going to work for his American uncle in Boston, and he wants Maureen to come with him as soon as she can. The letter also reveals that he was unable to perform sexually when they were together, but he tells her that it was only because he was drunk. He also tells her that there will be a going away party for him. He sends the letter to Ray, with explicit instructions to put it directly into Maureen's hands. However, when Ray comes to the house, Maureen is out, and Mag persuades him to leave the letter with her. After Ray leaves, Mag reads and burns the letter.

On the night of Pato's farewell party, Maureen is aware of Pato's plans but assumes he is uninterested in her because she wasn't invited. However, she tells Mag that it was she who broke it off with him. When Maureen keeps talking about sex, Mag teases her and accidentally says that she knows about Pato's impotence. Maureen understands that Mag must have read her letter, so she tortures Mag with hot oil until Mag confesses. Leaving Mag on the floor, Maureen gets dressed and rushes out to the party.

She returns home after midnight, telling an unmoving Mag that she caught Pato before he left, and they reaffirmed their relationship. At the end of the scene, Maureen bashes her mother's head in with a poker.

A month later, Mag's funeral is held following an investigation that cleared Maureen. Ray, Pato's brother, visits, bringing word from Pato. From their discussion, it becomes clear that Maureen imagined her reunion with Pato. He never saw Maureen before he left and is now engaged to a woman with whom he danced at the party. Maureen asks Ray to send Pato a message: "The beauty Queen of Leenane says 'Goodbye.'" All alone in the house, Maureen puts on Mag's sweater, sits in her chair, and uses her mannerisms.

This is a powerful and sad story that is largely inaccurate about mental illness. What mental illness could Maureen have? If it is depression, she wouldn't have the energy that she has. If it is psychosis, she wouldn't have such lucidity and be able to outsmart her mother the way she does. However, the mother-daughter relationship is realistic, illustrating two unhappy women torturing each other. I would say that the mother, Mag, has passive-aggressive personality disorder (PAPD). She is negative and basically passive in her aggression toward her daughter, Maureen. Mag burns letters, teases, and provides many impediments to Maureen's life. She cannot express her hostility toward her daughter directly. After all, she's supposed to be a loving mother. People exhibiting a passive-aggressive personality will often reply to an innocent comment sarcastically (if they respond at all). Individuals with PAPD won't smile or engage through eye contact; they will often remain silent, like Mag, and not say a word even when the people around them might be joking and laughing. Being with a person with PAPD is challenging to manage and often promotes feelings of sadness and anger. Maureen handled her mother the best she could, but then she lost it.

Maureen experiences her mother as punishing and manipulative, but she may just be dependent and self-detrimental. Mag is sulky, grumpy, gloomy, and moody. She may be depressed as well. Maureen killing Mag is totally unexpected, but when dealing with individuals with PAPD one may feel such rage and feel like destroying them.

The Marriage Proposal (1889) by Anton Chekhov concerns Ivan Vasilevich Lomov, a long-time neighbor of Stepan Stepanovich Chubukov, who has come to propose marriage to Chubukov's daughter, Natalia. After he has asked and received permission to marry Natalia, she is invited into the room, and he tries to propose. Lomov, while trying to make himself clear, gets into an argument with Natalia about a disputed piece of land between their respective properties. Since he is a hypochondriac, he gets palpitations and numbness in his leg while talking. After her father notices they are arguing, he joins in, and then sends Ivan out of the house. Her father Chubukov calls Lomov a fool that dared to make Natalia a proposal of marriage. Natalia then realizes that Lomov wanted to marry her and immediately has hysterics, begging for her father to bring him back. He does, and Natalia and Ivan get into a second big argument, this time about their dogs. Ivan collapses from his exhaustion over arguing, and father and daughter fear he's dead, sending them into another round of hysterics. However, after a few minutes Ivan regains consciousness, and Chubukov all but forces him and his daughter to seal the proposal with a kiss. Immediately following the kiss, the couple gets into another argument over their dogs while Chubukov tries to calm them and offers champagne.

This comedy illustrates Lomov as a person with PAPD who can't get to the point and who is aggressive and self-defeating.

10

Depression and Bipolar Disorder

Depression is a condition that most people think they understand. However, in psychiatry we have a specific definition. A person has to have five (or more) of these symptoms every day for at least two weeks: (1) depressed mood (sad, empty, hopeless); (2) decreased pleasure and interest in things; (3) significant weight loss (or decrease in appetite) or increase in appetite; (4) insomnia or hypersomnia; (5) agitation or slowing down; (6) fatigue or loss of energy; (7) feeling worthless or guilty; (8) decreased ability to think or concentrate; (9) recurrent thoughts of death.[1]

Night, Mother is a play by Marsha Norman that won the Pulitzer Prize for drama in 1983. A daughter, Jessie, and her mother, Thelma, have a dialogue about why Jessie wants to commit suicide. Obviously, Jessie has depression (as she has more than five of the symptoms mentioned above). Her mother and Jessie discuss Jessie's unhappy marriage and divorce, her criminal son, the loss of her father, and her epilepsy. Jessie says she is just tired of living. Thelma tries to reason with her, to no avail. At the end, Jessie shoots herself with her father's gun. Psychiatrists know that you probably can't talk a person out of suicide the way Thelma tried. The best way to deal with people who want to kill themselves is to hospitalize them.

Uncle Vanya, a famous play by Chekhov, was first produced in 1899 at the Moscow Art Theater. This was a time when Freud and his theories were popular. Konstantin Stanislavski was the director; Stanislavski is famous for his system of acting, in which actors attempt to get into the inner world or the psychological realism of the character. Stanislavski called this system the art of representation. He mobilized the actor's conscious thoughts and will with unconscious behavior. Stanislavski's method acting has been a staple of theater in New York. Three teachers—Lee Strasberg, Stella Adler, and Sanford Meisner—emphasized "the method." Marlon Brando and Robert De Niro are just a few of the famous actors who studied this method.

---

[1] American Psychiatric Association, *Diagnostic and Statistical Manual of Mental Disorders* (5th ed.) (Washington, DC: American Psychiatric Association, 2013).

In *Uncle Vanya*, an elderly professor, Serebryakov, and his second young, glamorous wife, Yelena, visit their rural estate. His friend, Astrov, is the local doctor. Maria is Vanya's mother. Sonya is the daughter of the professor's first wife. Vanya and Astrov fall in love with Yelena. Sonya loves Astrov but can't express it. Vanya complains about everything and eventually is able to get angry that the professor wants to sell the estate where he, his mother, and his niece Sonya all live. Vanya's a typical "paralyzed" depressive until he picks up a gun and tries to shoot the professor. He misses and wants to commit suicide by shooting himself instead. Nothing goes right for him. He can't sleep or eat well. He's sad most of the time or irritable. It's been nearly every day for longer than two weeks. He has diminished interest in things. He's agitated and wants to commit suicide. These are classical symptoms of major depression as defined in psychiatry. Chekhov was a doctor also and probably knew many depressives like Vanya in his career.

Vanya and Sonia and Misha and Spike is a hilarious comedy by Christopher Durang. Many of the show's elements were derived from *Uncle Vanya*, the *Cherry Orchard*, and *The Seagull*. In Durang's play, three middle-aged siblings fight and argue while Masha threatens to sell the house in rural Pennsylvania. Masha is an actress who supports Vanya and Sonia. They all bemoan their Chekhovian life. Spike is Masha's much younger lover. Masha tells them to dress up as Snow White characters. She will be Snow White, and they can be the Seven Dwarfs and go to a local party. Ben Brantley of the *New York Times* called this play "a sunny new play about gloomy people."[2] Yes, they are depressed like Chekhov's characters, but the play is so funny. I was laughing nonstop and forgetting to analyze these unfortunate people—not the way I felt during *Uncle Vanya*, which is depressing.

Coastal Disturbances by Tina Howe is a love story with depressed characters. Holly Dancer, the niece of M. J. Adams, an artist, comes to visit on a private beach in Massachusetts. Holly is attracted to the lifeguard Leo. Ariel Took is a divorced and depressed mother of Winston. The young people are absorbed in flirting and happiness, while Ms. Took tries to recover from her divorce. She is harsh and cruel to her son.

Many people with depression act the way Ms. Took does. They are unusually mean to other people because they are suffering from sadness,

[2] Brantley, Ben, "Insecure Namesakes With a Gloomy Worldview: Vanya and Sonia and Masha and Spike at Lincoln Center," *New York Times*, November 12, 2012.

hopelessness, and the other symptoms of depression. Many times after treatment, their harshness and cruelty lessen. People will feel like they are dealing with a different person after treatment.

Death of a Salesman by Arthur Miller premiered on Broadway in 1949. It has been presented many times. In 1949, it won both the Pulitzer Prize and the Tony Award for best play. Willy Loman, the salesman, is a tired man in his sixties. His wife, Linda, worries about him because she can see he's depressed. Their two sons, Biff and Happy, reminisce about their childhoods, but Biff failed math and can't get into college, even though he has potential as a football star. Willy's indecisiveness and daydreaming also disturb the boys. Willy's anger toward them causes them to make a business proposition to him. They all fail in their plans. Biff was turned off when he walked in on his father having an affair in Boston. Biff was disappointed in Willy, and that trauma caused him to alter the course of his life. Willy becomes psychotic, believing he is talking to his long-dead brother about his plan to kill himself and leave the insurance money to his family.

Willy has all the classical symptoms of depression. He's sad; he has anhedonia; he doesn't eat or sleep. He's so tired and guilty. His family experience him as angry. Willy seems to have a psychotic depression as well since he hears and sees his dead brother, Ben.

I was not surprised that Willy committed suicide. He—like many depressed patients—sees no way out of his problems. When a person suffers from depression, his thoughts are narrowed down into a dark tunnel. Depressed people actually have fewer neurotransmitters flowing through their brains, so that their thoughts are scanty and limited. Antidepressants, electroconvulsive therapy (ECT), and other brain stimulation techniques such as ketamine infusions all increase neurotransmission and bring relief to depressed patients. In 1949, when Miller wrote *Death of a Salesman*, we only had ECT as a treatment for depression.

The usual belief that clinical depression is something bizarre or foreign to most people is inaccurate. Depression strikes fifteen to thirty percent of adults at some point in their lives. Everyone has felt sad at times, and the familiarity of these feelings may allow depressed individuals to deny their illness. Willy was in denial about his depression, thinking that his lack of money and failures were the causes. Most people believe that if they are coping with a tragic event or difficult situation, they have a right to be depressed. Moreover, they think that their depression will be relieved as soon as the tragedy is alleviated, and that the depression is dependent on the event. This is untrue; if the depression is ongoing for six months, then that individual's brain chemistry may have changed and the person could be clinically depressed.

The inadequacy of the word *depression* becomes apparent here. Major depression, the kind that requires treatment, is different from the everyday blues people regularly experience.

Depression is one of the most common psychiatric disorders. Yet, because it is so common, many people feel that if they ignore the depression, it will disappear. If the condition reaches a clinical level, decreased or increased appetite and either insomnia or hypersomnia may develop. At this point, treatment is needed. Most people with depression also have a "blue" mood on a daily basis, anhedonia (loss of pleasure), either agitation or fatigue, poor concentration, increased self-criticism, and excessive guilt. If left untreated, depression may lead to suicide, as we see in *Death of a Salesman*. Suicide is a real threat in depression.

When I saw *Frankie and Johnny in the Clair de Lune* by Terrence McNally (1987), I was so saddened. Two lonely, middle-aged people on a first date wind up in her apartment on the West Side of Manhattan. Johnny is a short-order cook, and Frankie is a waitress. She believes she's unattractive because she's overweight and frumpy. But Johnny thinks she's his soulmate. The two reveal themselves to each other throughout the course of the play, and it's beautiful. At the end, they listen to Debussy's "Clair de lune" while looking at the moon.

Terrence McNally (1938–2020) has been described as the "bard of American theater." He was writing plays for years, but *Frankie and Johnny* made his career. In 1994, he presented *Love! Valour! Compassion!*—a play about the relationships between eight gay men. He himself was gay and out of the closet. This play won him his second Tony Award. When he wrote *Corpus Christi* (1997), many people protested because he retold Jesus's story and portrayed him and his disciples as a bunch of gay men. The religious right even put a death threat out on McNally!

Mothers and Sons (2014) is about a mother who lost her son to AIDS twenty years ago. She visits his partner, who in the meantime has married another man. The mother rejected her son because he was gay. She now has a chance to change her opinion of her son as she learns more about him from his lover. The mother is so sad from her loss, even though it is twenty years after his death in the play; but instead of deepening her emotions and mourning with the partner, she debates him. It's quite possible that McNally's own mother rejected him because he was gay, and that he had experienced similar conversations with her.

Sylvia (1995) by A. R. Gurney is about a middle-aged, upper-middle-class man, Greg, who finds Sylvia, a dog (played by a woman), in the park. He likes her so much that he brings her back to the empty nest he shares with Kate. When Kate gets home, she detests Sylvia and wants her gone. They eventually decide that Sylvia can stay for a few days before making a decision about her staying longer. Greg and Sylvia have already bonded. Over the next few days, Greg spends more and more time with Sylvia and less time at his job. Greg and Sylvia go on long walks, discussing life. Already dissatisfied with his job, Greg now has another reason to avoid work.

The conflict increases between Greg and Kate, who still does not like Sylvia. Eventually, Greg becomes completely obsessed with Sylvia, and Kate fears their marriage is breaking up. Kate and Sylvia are fighting with each other, each committed to seeing the other defeated. Greg meets a stranger at the dog run, who gives Greg tips on how to manage Sylvia and his predicament with Kate. When Greg has Sylvia spayed, Sylvia is angry and in pain, but she still loves him completely.

Kate's friend pays a visit and is repulsed by Greg and Sylvia. Greg and Kate visit a therapist, Leslie, who is sometimes male and sometimes female depending on her patients' state of mind. After a session with Greg, Leslie tells Kate to get a gun and shoot Sylvia.

Kate is asked to teach abroad, in London, and tells Greg that the English have a six-month quarantine for any dogs coming into the country. Greg is unwilling, but eventually he gives the news to Sylvia that he must give her away to a family who have a farm. Greg and Sylvia have a heated and tender moment. Kate and Sylvia say goodbye but, before Greg and Sylvia leave for the farm, Sylvia gives them the annotated and slightly chewed version of *All's Well That Ends Well* that Kate has been looking for, so Kate has a change of heart.

The last scene is directed toward the audience. Sylvia has died, and Greg and Kate still hold her memory in fondness.

Producers were hesitant to put this play on because *Sylvia* equated a dog and a woman and might be perceived as antifeminist. I believe that Gurney was attempting to show Greg as a depressed man who projected his love onto a dog and how he saw her as a person, as a woman. Greg was not getting enough love at home from Kate, who was preoccupied with her career. Once he brought Sylvia home, he was showing his wife that he needed more love from her to save himself. The play developed into a triangle between Greg, Kate, and Sylvia. Greg became obsessed with Sylvia. Many times depressed individuals will manifest obsessive features because both depression and obsessive-compulsive disorder (OCD) are the result of inadequate neurotransmission.

Obsessive-compulsive disorder features a pattern of unwanted thoughts and fears (obsessions) that lead a person to do repetitive behaviors (compulsions). These obsessions and compulsions interfere with daily activities and cause significant distress. Greg was distressed with his obsession with Sylvia, which compromised his marriage.

He tried to ignore or stop his obsessions, but that only increased his distress and anxiety.

Next to Normal (2009) by Brian Yorkey (book and lyrics) and Tom Kitt (music) is a musical about bipolar disorder. I was pleasantly surprised to see how well this disorder was dealt with. It starts off with Diana, a suburban mother who has bipolar disorder, up late waiting for the return of her son Gabe, who has broken curfew. Diana's daughter Natalie, an overachieving high school student studying for an upcoming test, is also awake. Diana wants her daughter to take a break and rest. Gabe gets home, and Diana's husband, Dan, wakes up to help the family prepare for the day. Diana makes an exaggerated meal for her family, but Dan and Natalie stop her when they realize she has made many more sandwiches than necessary. Dan takes care of Diana, while Natalie and Gabe leave for school.

At school, Natalie expresses her frustration as she practices for an upcoming piano recital in the music room. Henry, a classmate who loves Natalie from afar, enters. Meanwhile, Diana repeatedly visits her psychiatrist's office. She is prescribed too many medications, which all give her terrible side effects. Her faithful husband, Dan, waits through her appointments in the car. Diana finally gets a medication that numbs all feelings, and the doctor says she's stable.

Diana misses her old life when she felt things deeply. She resents her numbness with the new medications. She flushes her medications down the toilet at Gabe's suggestion.

Dan makes a family dinner so Henry can join them. When Diana brings a cake in for Gabe's birthday, Dan gently reminds her that Gabe died sixteen years ago. Diana has been hallucinating Gabe. Natalie freaks out and runs into her bedroom. Dan clears off the dinner table while Diana says she has stopped her medication. Dan begs her to let him help however he can since he's been there for her. Diana hallucinates Gabe then and rejects Dan. Natalie in her bedroom with Henry laments her mother's attachment to the dead Gabe. Diana hears their conversation and tells Natalie that she loves her as much as she can.

Diana visits a new doctor and does talk therapy and hypnosis. During the session, she sees Gabe, who asserts that he's still there. Diana says that she was unable to hold Natalie in the hospital when she was born. Natalie blows an important piano recital when she notices her parents are not there. Diana's doctor wants her to spend time with Natalie and let Gabe go. Diana goes home and cleans out some boxes of Gabe's things, but she sees Gabe again. He convinces her to commit suicide so they can be together.

Diana goes to the hospital after her suicide attempt. Her doctor tells Dan that they have to do ECT. Dan goes home to clean up Diana's mess. Natalie gets angry at her father to think that he has agreed to her mother's shock therapy. At the hospital, Diana has been fighting about the ECT, but she finally reluctantly agrees and signs the papers.

In act 2, Diana receives a series of ECT treatments. Natalie experiments with drugs and goes to clubs. Henry rescues Natalie many nights. When Diana returns home from the hospital, we discover that she has lost her memories of the last nineteen years. Henry gets rejected by Natalie when he asks her to go out. Dan learns that memory loss is a common side effect of ECT. Diana has even forgotten about Gabe, and Dan hesitates to remind her of him. After cleaning out boxes with her family, Diana is briefly confronted by Gabe, who reminds her that she has forgotten a vital part of her life.

At the doctor's, Diana is again inadvertently reminded of Gabe. Amazed, Diana returns home and searches through Gabe's old things. She finds his music box, which helped him sleep as a baby. Dan sees her and reminds her that their son died of an illness all the doctors missed. Diana admits she recalls hallucinating Gabe as a teenager, and Dan says they will do more ECT. They fight, and Natalie hears them. Natalie runs upstairs to Henry. Diana asks Dan about why he stays with her after all this. Dan is true to their wedding vows no matter what. Henry makes a pledge to Natalie in a similar vein. Diana, seeing Gabe again, pulls away from Dan.

Diana leaves Dan, goes to the doctor, and questions the doctor about why she can't get better. He recommends more shock treatment and medications, but she leaves him. Outside, she connects with Natalie for the first time. They embrace and agree that they will get a life somewhere "next to normal." Diana drives Natalie to the dance to meet Henry, where Natalie voices her concerns to Henry that she will someday end up like her mother. Henry promises to stand by her no matter what.

Diana returns home and tells Dan she is leaving him. She still loves him, but they must deal with their grief on their own. Dan looks back on his years of faithfulness to her and sees Gabe for the first time. The two embrace and Dan says Gabe's name for the first and only time in the show. Gabe disappears, and Natalie returns home to find that her mother is gone. She continues going out with Henry. Diana has moved in with her parents temporarily, still depressed but more hopeful than she's ever been. Dan visits her doctor, who gives him the name of another psychiatrist he can go to. Gabe is seen by the audience one final time, as hopeful and not threatening.

Every time I saw Diana hallucinating Gabe, I fell out of the story. In bipolar disorder, patients usually do not have visual hallucinations. They have auditory hallucinations mostly. I could accept this metaphor theoretically, but my knowledge as a psychiatrist prevented me from totally suspending my disbelief to enjoy the story. They didn't have to give Diana bipolar disorder. They could have just presented her as a grieving mother mourning her lost son. She could have had psychotic depression.

11

Psychosis

Although "psychosis" is a term that is thrown around loosely in everyday parlance, it has a specific meaning in psychiatry. I hear people casually saying that something or someone is "psychotic" to mean they are using extreme behavior or acting/behaving "far out" in some way. In psychiatry, psychotic means that a person has lost touch with reality. Usually, the person has hallucinations or delusions of some sort.

Schizophrenia involves psychosis in specific ways. Patients suffering from schizophrenia have problems with thinking, behavior, and emotions. Signs and symptoms may vary. Some definitions will be helpful.

Delusions are fixed and false beliefs that are not based in reality. For example, you may think that you're being harmed or harassed when you're clearly not. That would be considered paranoia and is quite common in psychosis. It is impossible to talk or reason anyone out of a delusion.

Hallucinations usually involve seeing or hearing things that don't exist. Yet for the person with schizophrenia, they seem as real as a normal experience. Hallucinations can be in any of the senses, but hearing voices is the most common hallucination. We call that auditory hallucinations.

Disorganized thinking may be inferred from disorganized speech. Effective communication can be impaired, and answers to questions may be completely unrelated. Rarely, speech may include putting together meaningless words that can't be understood, sometimes known as word salad.

Extremely disorganized or abnormal motor behavior may appear in a number of ways, from childlike silliness to unpredictable agitation. Behavior can include resistance to instructions, inappropriate or bizarre postures, a complete lack of response, or useless and excessive movement.

Negative symptoms refer to decreased ability or the lack of ability to function normally. For example, the person may neglect personal hygiene or appear to lack emotion. Also, the person may lose interest in everyday activities, socially withdraw, or lack the ability to experience pleasure.

In men, schizophrenia symptoms typically start in the early to mid-twenties. In women, symptoms typically begin in the late twenties. It's uncommon for children to be diagnosed with schizophrenia and rare for those older than age 45.

Schizophrenia symptoms in teenagers are similar to those in adults, but the condition may be more difficult to recognize. This may be in part because some of the early symptoms of schizophrenia in teenagers are common for typical development during teen years, such as withdrawal from friends and family, drop in performance at school, insomnia, irritability or depressed mood, and lack of motivation. Also, recreational substance use, such as marijuana, methamphetamines, or psychedelics, can sometimes cause similar signs and symptoms.

Bipolar disorder (formerly called manic-depressive illness or manic depression) is a mental disorder that causes unusual shifts in mood, energy, activity levels, concentration, and the ability to carry out day-to-day tasks.

There are three types of bipolar disorder. All three types involve clear changes in mood, energy, and activity levels. These moods range from periods of extremely "up," elated, irritable, or energized behavior (known as manic episodes) to very "down," sad, indifferent, or hopeless periods (known as depressive episodes). Less severe manic periods are known as hypomanic episodes.

Bipolar I disorder is defined by manic episodes that last at least seven days or by manic symptoms that are so severe that the person needs immediate hospital care. Usually, depressive episodes occur as well, typically lasting at least two weeks. Episodes of depression with mixed features (having depressive symptoms and manic symptoms at the same time) are also possible.

Bipolar II disorder is defined by a pattern of depressive episodes and hypomanic episodes, but not the full-blown manic episodes that are typical of bipolar I disorder.

Cyclothymic disorder (also called cyclothymia) is defined by periods of hypomanic symptoms as well as periods of depressive symptoms lasting for at least two years (one year in children and adolescents). However, the symptoms do not meet the diagnostic requirements for a hypomanic episode and a depressive episode.

Bipolar disorder is usually diagnosed during late adolescence or early adulthood. Occasionally, bipolar symptoms can appear in children. Bipolar disorder can also first appear during a woman's pregnancy or following childbirth. Although the symptoms may vary over time, bipolar disorder usually requires lifelong treatment. Following a prescribed treatment plan can help people manage their symptoms and improve their quality of life.

People with bipolar disorder experience periods of unusually intense emotion, changes in sleep patterns and activity levels, and uncharacteristic behaviors. These distinct periods are called "mood episodes." Mood episodes are very different from the moods and behaviors that are typical for the person. During an episode, the symptoms last every day for most of the day. Episodes may also last for longer periods, such as several days or weeks.

Rarely do we see truly psychotic characters portrayed correctly in plays. Playwrights may hint at extreme mental illness in one of their characters, but to show psychosis accurately is rare. One play, *The House of Blue Leaves* (by John Guare, 1971), does an excellent job of showing the psychosis of Bananas, Artie's wife, since she has schizophrenia. She is headed for a mental hospital, which is referred to euphemistically as "the house of blue leaves." The play is set in Queens, 1965, on the day Pope Paul VI visited New York City. Artie, a songwriter and zookeeper, wants to take his girlfriend, Bunny, to Hollywood. The play is known for "smart comic lunacy."[1]

I felt great sympathy for Bananas when I saw the play in 1986. Bananas is being fooled by Artie so that he can escape from her with his girlfriend. It's supposed to be good fun, but I cringe whenever mental illness is the butt of jokes. However, the depiction of Bananas as completely out of touch with reality and probably hallucinating was realistic.

Proof (2000) by David Auburn is about Catherine, the daughter of the deceased Robert, a math genius, who developed a proof of prime numbers. Robert became psychotic. He was concerned with decoding extraterrestrial messages as well as probably hallucinating. His daughter Catherine is left trying to prove her father's proofs. She fears that she will become psychotic like her father.

Too often, genius and mental illness are paired with each other. Usually, a genius (e.g., Vincent Van Gogh, Alan Turing, Leo Tolstoy) creates *in spite of* his mental illness. Perhaps being psychotic, depressed, anxious, or any of the possible psychiatric problems allows a person to view the world in a unique way and thus create art, math, literature, and more.

Being psychotic is a huge burden. Not knowing what we all agree is "reality" and what is a delusion or a hallucination places a psychotic person in a precarious position. One would think that more playwrights would use psychotic characters because authors know they should keep their characters in danger at all times to write a thrilling play.

---

[1] Stasio, Marilyn, "Review: 'The House of Blue Leaves,'" *Variety*, April 25, 2011.

The Glass Menagerie by Tennessee Williams is often thought to be about how Tom, a stand-in for the playwright, dealt with his sister Laura's mental illness. In real life, Williams had a sister who suffered from schizophrenia. It's not clear from the play, which I've seen several times, if Laura has schizophrenia, autism, obsessive-compulsive disorder, or just agoraphobia. Williams's real sister Rose was subjected to a lobotomy. In the play, Amanda (Tom and Laura's mother) is anxious to marry Laura off, denying the extent of her daughter's mental illness. She pressures Tom to find a "gentleman caller" for Laura. When he finds Jim and brings him home, Laura withdraws into herself and her "glass menagerie." Laura is too mentally ill to be reacting to a gentleman caller. It turns out that Jim is engaged to someone else anyway, which angers Amanda, who put so much hope into him. Tom eventually leaves home, like Williams did, unable to deal with all the denial of reality in his family.

George Bernard Shaw wrote *Saint Joan* in 1923 about Joan of Arc, who was canonized by the Catholic Church a few years before he wrote his play. Joan is a simple peasant who sees visions of St. Margaret, St. Catherine, and Archangel Michael. She claims God sent her these visions. Of course, people around her are skeptical, especially Robert de Baudricourt, whom she asks for troops to go to Orleans. When his chickens lay eggs after a dry period without them, he begins to believe her and that she has special powers that will be useful to him. She is then received in the court of the weak and narcissistic dauphin, to whom she reveals that he will be king, and she'll rally his troops to drive out the English. She has Dunois lay siege to Orleans. The English—Warwick and Stogumber—can't believe that she's so successful, so they label her a witch and want to kill her. The dauphin is crowned Charles VII at Reins. Joan tries to take Paris, but then is captured. There is an ecclesiastical trial for her in which she's accused of heresy. She says her voices are from God, and she doesn't need Church officials. The church people hate this and condemn her to death at the stake because she doesn't want to be imprisoned. The bishop of Beauvais excommunicates her and gives her to the English, who burn her alive. Twenty-five years later, she's exonerated and cleared of heresy.

Joan is seen as a rebel against church authority and the feudal system. Psychiatry would see her as a woman with psychosis. Seeing visions and hearing voices happen most often in cases of bipolar disorder. Many of those afflicted see and hear things. Many times, they are extremely charismatic and lead people on all kinds of missions, like Joan. People with schizophrenia usually do not have visual hallucinations, but they can have auditory ones.

August Wilson's *Fences* is about race relations in Pittsburgh, Pennsylvania, and is set in the 1950s. A Black baseball league player, Troy, is now a garbage man. He lives a menial, respectable working-class life with his wife, Rose, and their teenager, Cory. Troy's younger brother, Gabe, is an ex-soldier with a war injury to his head. Gabe only got $3,000 for his injury, and Troy took control of it to buy his home for his family. The play begins with Troy talking and drinking with his coworker. His son, Cory, wants to go to college on a football scholarship, but Troy discourages him, saying that's not a good idea for a Black man. Eventually, Troy kicks Cory out of the house after they argue. Cory joins the Army. Troy admits to Rose that he has a mistress who is now pregnant. Rose will take the baby when it's born (and the mistress dies), but she kicks Troy out. When Troy dies seven years later, Cory comes back and at first refuses to go to Troy's funeral, but eventually does, and the family is reunited. There is forgiveness and redemption.

Gabriel, Troy's brother, is "crazy" due to his head injury. He symbolizes an angel. He wears a trumpet around his neck, chases "hell-hounds," and thinks he's talking to St. Peter. Like Joan of Arc, his psychosis is seen as a blessing from heaven. Mental patients have been either seen as innocents like this or portrayed as demons, witches, or "possessed" throughout history. Society has projected many things on the "insane" because most people could not understand mental illnesses. Even now, when we know schizophrenia, bipolar disorder, depression, and anxiety are caused by chemical imbalances and brain structure abnormalities, we still think of the mentally ill as ill in a different way than if they have other physical disorders.

Frozen (not to be confused with the musical with the same name), a play by Bryony Lavery, is about a serial killer, Ralph, who kidnaps a young girl, rapes, and kills her. A New York psychiatrist, Agnetha, travels to England to examine Ralph. The girl's mother, Nancy, interacts with Agnetha and Ralph until all the characters change and become "unfrozen." Forgiveness is the theme.

In this play, the psychiatrist is portrayed as rigid and frozen in her ways. When she really learns what causes Ralph to kill, it unlocks something in her. All the other characters learn about themselves in significant ways. Even the serial killer must face his psychosis. Here it is important to mention that the playwright was accused of plagiarism for this play, but Ms. Lavery proved she had used actual cases to write her story and thus had not plagiarized anyone. She wrote Ralph's part so well, the media couldn't believe she had made it up.

Jumpers, a play by Tom Stoppard, has meant many different things to many different people. Some critics called it "a shallow, display of pyrotechnics," and others thought it a brilliant display. George is a foolish philosophy professor at a university where the vice chancellor wants his faculty to exercise. One professor is shot dead during a chaotic opening scene, which causes a philosophical consideration of human morality. George's wife, Dotty, has some mental disorder that was caused by seeing men land on the moon. At the end, George shoots his pet rabbit dead, trying to demonstrate Zeno's paradox, and then he crushes the tortoise in his grief.

Dotty's psychosis is caused by taking the moon away from her as a metaphor. In other words, her delusions are shattered, but instead of helping her become sane, it causes her insanity—the opposite of how we psychiatrists see things.

Blue/Orange (2000) by Joe Penhall is a play that took place in a London mental hospital in which a mysterious patient claimed to be the son of an exiled African dictator. It seems more and more likely as the play unfolds that he was. Mr. Penhall was making the point that more Black men are given the diagnosis of schizophrenia than white men, and more of them are held against their will in mental hospitals. Supposedly one percent of our population has schizophrenia, without regard to race or gender. I have heard it said that if you are rich, you get the diagnosis of bipolar disorder, but if you are poor, you may be labeled schizophrenic. I haven't seen that in hospitals and clinics I've worked in, but many times it takes years before it becomes clear if a patient is cycling from mania to depression and back again (bipolar disorder), or if the patient just has episodes of psychosis without depression and is schizophrenic.

The Curious Incident of the Dog in the Nighttime (2013) was adapted by Simon Stephens from the novel by Mark Haddon. The story concerns a mystery surrounding the death of a neighbor's dog; the death is investigated by young Christopher Boone, who is autistic. We see how Christopher struggles in his relationships with his parents and school mentor. The play received a generally warm reception, with most critics impressed by its ability to convey the point of view of the young man and the compassion of his school mentor. Critics also generally spoke highly of the visual effects employed during the show.

Set in Swindon and London, the story concerns a fifteen-year-old amateur detective named Christopher, who is a mathematical genius. He appears to have an unspecified disorder that is variously described as either autism or Asperger syndrome, although the condition is never explicitly stated in the play. The titular curious incident is the mystery surrounding the death of a neighbor's dog, Wellington, found speared by a sharp garden fork.

While searching for the murderer of the dog, he encounters resistance from many neighbors, but mostly from his father, Ed. Christopher argues to himself that many rules are made to be broken, so he continues to search for an answer; he compares himself to Sherlock Holmes. When he discovers that his father had both lied about his mother being dead for several years and that he had killed Wellington, Christopher is distraught and fears for his own life. For the first time, he travels alone to London to find and live with his mother. He finds the journey overstimulating and stressful, but succeeds and is welcomed by his mother. However, his ambitions lead him back home, where he wants to sit for an A-level mathematics exam. Christopher achieves the best possible result and gradually reconciles with his father.

In a short scene after the curtain call, Christopher reappears to brilliantly solve his favorite question from the mathematics exam, which was so advanced that I had to buy the novel to understand the explanation.

Asperger syndrome is a condition on the autism spectrum, with generally higher functioning individuals. Patients with this condition may be socially awkward and have an all-absorbing interest in specific topics, as Christopher does. In the past, before this diagnosis became common parlance, people may have considered individuals with Asperger syndrome to be psychotic or even retarded.

Communication training and behavioral therapy can help people with the syndrome learn to socialize more successfully.

12

Substance Abuse

In Eugene O'Neill's *Long Day's Journey Into Night*, Mary, who is addicted to morphine, is the mother and center of a dysfunctional family where drinking is a problem. The two sons are Jamie and Edmund, who steal their father's (James's) alcohol. The father is a has-been actor, narcissistic, and miserly. Instead of being concerned with their own problems, everyone is worried that Mary will return to her addiction. She has just been discharged from a rehab center at the beginning of the play. Mary goes with her maid, Cathleen, to the drugstore and picks up her prescription for morphine. Edmund has tuberculosis, and all the men get drunk and fight. At the end, Mary, high on morphine, comes down with her wedding gown and rambles on about her love for her husband, as well as her convent days.

Morphine, which is a natural product of the opium poppy, sends its users into a totally tranquilized state where nothing matters, into a waking sleep where no problems exist. Many of the individuals who are addicted to opiates, which include morphine, suffered terrible abuse in their childhoods. Their abuse might have been mental, emotional, and/or physical. We are not sure what abuse, if any, Mary may have suffered, but she is addicted to morphine. Morphine was widely prescribed for pain when O'Neill wrote this play. Heroin was derived later from morphine and was originally designed to be nonaddictive, which of course it is not. Morphine and heroin are absorbed at the opiate receptors of the brain, where the natural opiates of the body, endorphins, are also absorbed. These opiate receptors regulate pain. The past abuse that morphine and heroin addicts experienced may have caused damage or some malfunctioning of the opiate receptor system. Through drug use, the addict may be trying to regulate his or her system. It could be that endorphins are insufficient, and the abuser adds artificial opiates (i.e., morphine or heroin) to modulate his or her malfunctioning. This is the theory of self-medication. "Junkies" tend to feel unworthy, but when they take heroin, they place themselves into a world where they no longer need to contend with adequacy issues. Unlike the cocaine users who inflate their self-image with their drug, heroin users float away to where image and worth no longer matter.

People with substance abuse may be considered to have a disability. Drug abuse is considered a disability or disease by the medical profession. Mary certainly is disabled by her addiction, but we don't view her the way we would if she had a physical disability, like blindness or paralysis. We tend to blame people with substance abuse for their addictions. If only they would stop and become sober. Of course, it is difficult for the addict to get clean and sober. Many programs have been developed to help those with drug abuse. Alcoholics Anonymous, AA, the worldwide fellowship of sobriety seekers, is the most effective path to abstinence according to many researchers.

After evaluating many studies, psychiatric investigators determined that AA was nearly always found to be more effective than psychotherapy in achieving abstinence. In addition, most studies showed that AA participation lowered healthcare costs.

Alcoholics Anonymous works because it's based on social interaction. AA members give each other emotional support as well as practical tips to refrain from drinking.

Alcohol is still the most popular drug in the United States and the one people don't consider a drug. In some cultures, it is necessary to drink alcohol to prove yourself. Alcoholics tend to find jobs where alcohol is free flowing, becoming waiters, waitresses, bartenders, and similar occupations. This does not mean that every bartender is an alcoholic, but alcoholics will look for an environment filled with their drug.

Addiction to alcohol is due to a complicated array of factors, including genetic predisposition and environmental attitudes. It has been found that the sons of alcoholics metabolize alcohol differently from the sons of nonalcoholics. They are able to tolerate larger doses of alcohol without feeling inebriated. The alcoholic tends to be a "people pleaser," an AA term. This is also consistent with the alcoholic as a dependent personality and one with many unresolved oral features. Low frustration tolerance and inability to deal with anger and other intense feelings are part of the psychological makeup of the alcoholic.

Addiction is a primary, chronic, neurobiological disease with genetic, psychosocial, and environmental factors, characterized by behaviors of impaired control over use, compulsive use, continued use despite harm, and craving. Some consider it an operantly conditioned response to a substance, with the response becoming stronger as time goes on.

The Marriage of Bette and Boo (1985) by Christopher Durang deals with their marriage, stillbirths, divorce, and alcoholism. The play follows the heartbreaking marriage of Bette Brennan and Boo Hudlocke. Bette and Boo marry and get ready to have a large, happy family that Bette always dreamed of. Bette has a succession of stillbirths. Bette is devastated, and Boo starts to drink. Bette nags him. Both of them deal with their impossible families. Bette's father had a stroke and only speaks in unintelligible gibberish. Boo's sadistic father calls his long-suffering the father's wife "the dumbest woman in the world." Bette's sister has so much anxiety, she finds it necessary to apologize for everything. It's been thought that this play is Durang's most autobiographical work. Three decades of marriage are covered in thirty-three scenes. We don't get into any depth regarding the characters, but we understand them in their context. Boo's alcoholism may be the cause of Bette's stillbirths. The alcoholism definitely fuels the fights Bette and Boo have.

Theresa Rebeck's *The Scene* opens with a Manhattan party where Clea, an attractive twenty-something Ohioan, is conversing with two men, Charlie, a middle-aged, washed-up actor, and Lewis. Clea talks in "Valley Girl" about how weird New York City is. She's showing herself off as beautiful but dumb and claims she doesn't drink due to genetic alcoholism. Later she accepts Lewis's vodka offer. After drinking the vodka, Clea goes into a rant about this new job she has which is a void. She also rants about her boss, Stella, calling her an infertile "Nazi priestess," obsessed with her job and her baby adoption process. Stella turns out to be Charlie's wife.

Stella, Charlie, and Lewis are drinking at Stella and Charlie's apartment, listening to Stella's rant about Clea, calling her an idiot who can barely speak English but looks good from the back. Lewis is sent out to get drinks, and Stella complains about how miserable she is at work. Charlie then goes on a rant about the party. Stella asks Charlie if he spoke to Nick, Charlie's arch nemesis. Nick and Charlie went to high school together.

Clea first dates Lewis, soon moving to Charlie. His wife catches them in the act, and Charlie is unable to resolve the situation. He loses his wife—Lewis is happy to console her—Clea drops him and moves on, and all he has left is his bottle and his misery.

Post-traumatic stress disorder (PTSD) may be caused by witnessing or experiencing a traumatic event. Those experiencing PTSD, many of whom may be veterans or the survivors of a natural disaster or violent act, might turn to drugs or alcohol to self-medicate feelings of fear, anxiety, and stress. People have involuntary and intrusive thoughts, distressing dreams, dissociation, physiological reactions (exaggerated startle response or trouble sleeping). They may try to avoid situations that remind them of the trauma. It's not surprising that they would resort to drugs or alcohol to escape this condition.

Most people who have suffered through traumatic events eventually overcome the anxiety and depression caused by those experiences. But when PTSD develops, these symptoms don't just go away. They might last for months or years after the event.

Following a traumatic experience, the brain produces fewer endorphins, one of the chemicals that help us feel good. People with PTSD may turn to alcohol and other mood-enhancing drugs, which increase endorphin levels. Over time, they may come to rely on drugs to relieve all of their feelings of depression, anxiety, and irritability.

Water by the Spoonful by Quiara Alegria Hudes (2011) is the second part of a trilogy: *Elliot: A Soldier's Fugue.* In the first part, a young marine, Elliot, comes to terms with his time in Iraq and his father's and grandfather's time in Viet Nam and Korea, respectively. *Water* takes place seven years later, after Elliot has returned to his home in Philadelphia. He's been wounded and works in a sandwich shop. At night he cares for Ginny, his sick aunt, who raised him. He has PTSD and is dealing with it the best he can. He sees a ghost who offers a hand and repeats an Arabic phrase. He asks Professor Aman to translate the phrase and gets involved in doing a documentary about the Iraq War. Odessa, Elliot's birth mother and a sister to Ginny, runs an anonymous message board for recovering addicts. Ginny dies and leaves Elliot with little funds to bury her. Elliot confronts his mother, Odessa, about the fact that she let his little sister die and refused to give her "water by the spoonful," which she needed to survive because his mother was too busy getting high on crack cocaine. Elliot pawns his mother's computer to pay for the funeral. Odessa relapses and overdoses. Elliot and his cousin scatter Ginny's ashes in Puerto Rico, and Elliot plans to go to Los Angeles to act.

August: Osage County (2007) by Tracy Letts introduces us to Beverly Weston, a once-famous poet, interviewing Johnna, a Cheyenne woman, for a job as a live-in cook and caregiver for his wife, Violet, at the opening of the play. Violet had mouth cancer because she was a heavy smoker most of her life; in addition, she's an alcoholic addicted to drugs. She has terrible mood swings, but it's not clear if this mood-swing problem is due to her substance abuse or if she had an underlying psychiatric disorder to begin with. Beverly admits he is also an alcoholic. He hires Johnna and gives her a book of T. S. Elliot poems. Beverly disappears in the first act. The family learns his boat is missing. Violet tries to track him down, but in between drinking and drugging, she insults her own family: her daughter, Ivy; sister, Mattie Fay; and Mattie Fae's husband, Charlie. Another of Violet's daughters, Barbara, comes with her daughter, Jean (14 years old), and husband, Bill. She hasn't seen her mother for years. The 14-year-old Jean bonds with the caregiver, Johnna, after they smoke marijuana. They all hear that Beverly has drowned at the end of act 1. In act 2, they go to Beverly's funeral. Violet keeps popping pills and blaming her late husband. The third daughter, Karen, flies in from Florida with her new fiancé—Steve, a lecher. They have a memorial dinner, but Violet insults everyone. Barbara winds up physically attacking her mother for revealing her separation from Bill. Barbara orders the family to search the house for Violet's stash of drugs. After they calm down, the three sisters—Ivy, Barbara, Karen—discuss their mother, Violet. Other relationships are threatened during the course of the play. Barbara drinks heavily like her mother. Then, her sister Ivy accuses Barbara of turning into a Violet. Ivy is in love with her first cousin, Little Charles (who she thinks is Mattie Fae's son). She tries to keep it a secret, which is impossible in this dysfunctional family. It turns out that Little Charles is actually Beverly's son, which is worse because that would make him her brother! Violet blames Barbara for her husband's suicide. Violet's whole family leaves disgusted with her. Only Johnna is left, and she quotes T. S. Elliot: "This is the way the world ends, this is the way the world ends."

This play won a Pulitzer, a Tony, and a Drama Desk Award. Everyone loved this story of a sprawling Oklahoma family getting in trouble with each other every single minute. Nearly every imaginable tragic situation was dealt with in this complex play: alcoholism, drug addiction, racism, infidelity, and incest.

The alcoholism and drug addiction of Violet and her husband, Beverly, begin the difficulties of this family. Perhaps Violet had bipolar disorder or an anxiety disorder before she began using addictive substances. We psychiatrists call this a dual diagnosis when a person has a psychiatric diagnosis along with a drug or alcohol addiction. Sometimes it's like the old cliché of which came first: the chicken or the egg. Often, we can't tell, but in psychiatry we first detox the patient from the drugs and alcohol. Then we try to determine what other possible mental conditions could be lurking underneath those addictions. Is it bipolar disorder? Or is it depression, anxiety, or panic attacks? Then, we treat the patients with the appropriate medications.

Many times, we consider alcohol or drugs to be self-medication of the wrong kind.

Halfway Bitches Go Straight to Heaven (2019) by Stephen Adly Guirgis. The play takes place in a rundown halfway house for women on New York's Upper West Side. In three hours, we see an assembly of many addicted and struggling characters in short, episodic scenes. Announcements are made of such activities as an "Incest Survivors Meeting" and a "You, Me, and Hepatitis C" workshop that the residents can attend.

They're an emotionally troubled group of women with Happy Meal Sonia and her devoted adult daughter, Taina, as well as the tough-as-nails war veteran Sarge, who loves the single mom and former stripper, Bella. There's an elegant Wanda Wheels, a former actress in a wheelchair, who regales the others with stories of her past, including having once dated Noam Chomsky; an obese Betty Woods, a self-published author of erotic fiction; the smelly Queen Sugar, desperately attempting to improve her finances via an Amway-style pyramid scheme dubbed "Fam-Way"; and Venus, a trans woman targeted by Sarge, among others, because they consider her a man who shouldn't be taking up space in a home for women.

The staff includes the African-born Mr. Mobo, who can't resist the seduction of the sexually aggressive resident Munchies. Joey, a married custodian who finds himself falling in love with Venus; social worker, Jennifer, whose well-heeled upbringing and style of dressing alienate the residents; and the beleaguered head of the facility, Miss Rivera, who alleviates her frustrations by drinking vodka in her coffee cup. It's a habit she shares with Wanda Wheels, who similarly spikes her Ensure. Another regular presence is Father Miguel, the sort of urban priest equally capable of delivering thoughtful counseling or violently subduing an abusive husband who periodically shows up demanding to see his wife.

There's a lot going on in this drama, but the major plot points include the mysterious disappearance of one of the residents and an episode involving a stolen goat that suffers a terrible end. Toward the conclusion, the playwright makes a compelling point about society's misplaced priorities with the introduction of a detective and politician's aide who show up at the halfway house, not to investigate the case of the missing resident, but rather that of the purloined goat.

The sheer plethora of social ills on display, including drug addiction, alcoholism, sexual abuse, mental illness, domestic abuse, PTSD, and governmental indifference to the lower rungs of society, proves a bit overwhelming.

Guirgis, who usually writes with a tighter focus, has trouble keeping all of his narrative balls in the air, with the result that while some characters and plot elements are vividly rendered, others are given short shrift and make little impression.

Emma, the protagonist in Duncan Macmillan's *People, Places and Things* (2015), suffers a lot, but she is amused by how far and fast she can fall and still pull back before landing at the bottom. Like many junkies, Emma is a sentimental mess, chasing the dragon with coke and alcohol. She also chases love, which involves regret as well. She would only connect if she could or if that held her interest.

Emma's an actress, a druggy narcissist in a world of them. She is an exhibitionist, and the audience is her voyeur. Onstage, she works her way through failed dreams and unrequited love. We are reminded of Chekhov's *The Seagull*. Is Emma Nina with her unfulfilled dreams? Emma says, "I'm a seagull," but the words are indistinct as she nods off, here and there. The scene changes, and Emma goes off to a rave in a club with party people who don't want the night to end.

The next day—or some other day—Emma sits, stoned in the lobby of a rehab facility in London. She's on the phone with someone—we don't know whom at first. She's asking the person to clean out her apartment and get rid of all the hidden pills and bottles, which most addicts do when they first get sober. She says, in between twitching and twisting, that the person should listen to her. Who is she speaking to so agonizingly? Of course, it's her mother, who never listened to her in the first place. It sounds like her family and friends are revolting against her narcissism.

By seeking help, Emma puts us on her side. We all want to be rehabilitated, to be cleansed, and to be better. Emma needs to go through rehab if she's ever going to be hired as an actress again. Her desire to act is never far from her. She signs into rehab as "Nina."

We want to create new neural networks by watching plays. When we see plays that portray drug and alcohol addictions, we view characters who are trapped in their destructive and repetitive behaviors of addiction. These characters are not creating new networks; they are painfully reiterating their old patterns that cause them so many problems. Tension and conflict are paramount as they struggle to be free and perhaps transfer to a different pathway.

13

Identity Issues

Most characters in good plays establish their identities early on. The audience needs to be able to relate to the people on stage to enjoy the play. Shakespeare was a master at allowing his audience to identify with his characters. You quickly understand who everyone is in *Hamlet* and what they want, or in *Macbeth*, *King Lear*, and *Othello* as well. We also know who the people are in O'Neill's *Anna Christie* or *Desire Under the Elms*.

The identity of a character includes who the person is in terms of what values they hold, how they see themselves, their roles in society, their memories, experiences, and relationships. Usually, this combination of being in the world is steady over time and establishes their identity. We particularly appreciate when characters change during the course of the play. In fact, many times the hero or heroine of the story, the protagonist, is the person who changes the most—for better or worse.

In *Joe Egg* by Peter Nichols, a young couple, Bri and Sheila, deal with their daughter's disability. The girl, "Joe Egg" or Josephine, has cerebral palsy. Caring for her has defined who Bri and Sheila are. Joe Egg has occupied every minute of their lives since her birth. Bri, a schoolteacher, is handling it with humor, alcohol, and denial. Sheila is escaping the best she can with theater. And Joe Egg is herself at the center of their world, unable to escape her fate. The couple flirt but avoid sex throughout the play, perhaps because sex had brought them Joe Egg. They think they are being punished by having such a child. At the end, Bri almost kills their child and is ready to escape their life together, but Sheila brings him back into the family with sex. Maybe they can make another, healthier child. By having everything revolve around Joe Egg, the playwright gives the characters brilliant definitions of themselves.

The Merchant of Venice is structured like a comedy but has some dark spots and bitterness. Supposedly written in 1596–1597, a few years before *Twelfth Night* and *Measure for Measure*, it looks like a mature work. The play owes its maturity to the character of Shylock, whom Jews detest. Shylock goes beyond the play in terms of complexity. Was Shylock having a crisis of identity?

Antonio, the eponymous merchant of Venice, is sad because Bassanio, his closest friend, wants to marry Portia, and Antonio knows he will be left lonely when Bassanio marries. Bassanio needs a lot of money to become a suitor since he squandered his extensive estate. He asks Antonio for the money. Antonio agrees to give him the money, but he doesn't have the cash—he has ships and merchandise at sea. Bassanio goes to Shylock, a Jewish money-lender, and names Antonio as the guarantor. Shylock dislikes Antonio, who is anti-Semitic, and Antonio loans money without interest, forcing Shylock to charge less. Shylock doesn't want to give the loan, and he will take a pound of flesh if Antonio can't repay it on the given date.

Bassanio doesn't want Antonio to accept such a risky condition. Antonio signs the contract anyway. With money in hand, Bassanio leaves for Belmont with his friend Gratiano, a talkative young man.

Meanwhile, in Belmont, Portia has many suitors. Her father left a will that says that each of her suitors must choose correctly from one of three caskets, made of gold, silver, and lead, respectively. Whoever picks the right casket wins Portia's hand. The first suitor, the Prince of Morocco, chooses the gold casket. The second suitor, the conceited prince of Aragon, chooses the silver casket. Both suitors leave empty-handed, having rejected the lead casket because of the baseness of its material and its slogan: "Who chooseth me must give and hazard all he hath." The last suitor is Bassanio, whom Portia wishes to succeed, having met him before. As Bassanio ponders his choice, members of Portia's household sing a song to encourage him. Bassanio chooses the lead casket and wins Portia's hand.

At Venice, Antonio's ships are reported lost at sea, so the merchant cannot repay the bond. Shylock has become more determined to exact revenge from Christians because his daughter, Jessica, eloped with the Christian Lorenzo and converted. She took a substantial amount of Shylock's wealth with her. Shylock has Antonio brought before the court.

At Belmont, Bassanio receives a letter telling him that Antonio has been unable to repay the loan from Shylock. Portia and Bassanio marry. Bassanio and Gratiano leave for Venice, with money from Portia, to save Antonio's life by offering the money to Shylock. Unknown to Bassanio and Gratiano, Portia sent her servant, Balthazar, to seek the counsel of Portia's cousin, Bellario, a lawyer.

The climax of the play is set in the court of the duke of Venice. Shylock refuses Bassanio's offer of 6,000 ducats, twice the amount of the loan. He demands his pound of flesh from Antonio. The duke, wishing to save Antonio but unable to nullify a contract, refers the case to Balthazar, a young male "doctor of the law," bearing a letter of recommendation to the duke from the lawyer, Bellario. The doctor is Portia in disguise, and the law clerk who accompanies her is Nerissa, also disguised as a man. As Balthazar, Portia, in a famous speech, keeps asking Shylock to show mercy. However, Shylock adamantly refuses any compensations and insists on the pound of flesh.

As the court grants Shylock his bond and Antonio prepares for Shylock's knife, Portia deftly appropriates Shylock's argument for "specific performance." She says that the contract allows Shylock to remove only the flesh, not the blood, of Antonio. Thus, if Shylock were to shed any drop of Antonio's blood, his "lands and goods" would be forfeited under Venetian laws. She tells him that he must cut precisely one pound of flesh, no more, no less, or he will lose everything.

Defeated, Shylock consents to accept Bassanio's offer of money for the defaulted bond: to pay "the bond thrice," which Portia rejects, telling him to take his bond and then merely the principal; Portia also prevents him from doing this on the ground that he has already refused it "in the open court." She cites a law under which Shylock, as a Jew and therefore an "alien," having attempted to take the life of a citizen, has forfeited his property, half to the government and half to Antonio, leaving his life at the mercy of the duke. The duke spares Shylock's life and says he may remit the forfeiture. Portia says the duke may waive the state's share, but not Antonio's. Antonio says he is content that the state waive its claim to half Shylock's wealth if he can have his one-half share until Shylock's death, when the principal would be given to Lorenzo and Jessica. Antonio also asks that "for this favor" Shylock convert to Christianity and bequeath his entire estate to Lorenzo and Jessica. The duke then threatens to recant his pardon of Shylock's life unless he accepts these conditions. Shylock, rethreatened with death, accepts.

Bassanio does not recognize his disguised wife, but offers to give a present to the supposed lawyer. First, she declines, but after he insists, Portia requests his ring and Antonio's gloves. Antonio parts with his gloves without a second thought, but Bassanio gives the ring only after much persuasion from

Antonio, as earlier in the play he promised his wife never to lose, sell, or give it. Nerissa, as the lawyer's clerk, succeeds in likewise retrieving her ring from Gratiano, her husband, who also does not see through her disguise.

At Belmont, Portia and Nerissa taunt and pretend to accuse their husbands before revealing they were really the lawyer and his clerk in disguise. The other characters make amends, and Antonio learns that his ships are safe after all.

Antonio identifies himself by his friendship with Bassanio, whom he loses when that friend pursues Portia for marriage. He almost loses his life when Shylock is ready to cut off a pound of flesh. He is saved by Portia, who becomes a male lawyer, another transformation of identity. Her maid, Nerissa, is also disguised as a man, her identity change. Then there is poor Shylock, who loses all his wealth and his identity as a Jew. Shakespeare was cruel to punish Shylock in this way. Antisemitism was rampant in England at this time, and Shakespeare was no exception in regard to his prejudices. Most Jewish people are horrified by *The Merchant of Venice* and its portrayal of Jewish people.

Currently, people are having identity crises when they believe they have been born into the wrong sex. Since transsexual operations are so much more available today, males who feel they are really females and females who believe they are actually males may have themselves surgically altered to conform to their inner identities. Some people must have felt like this throughout history, but they had to suppress and hide their true feelings since society was not ready for their transformations. Perhaps Shakespeare constantly disguising females as males and males as females in his plays fulfilled some of society's unconscious wishes. Also, our medical procedures are so advanced at this point that we can surgically alter genitalia and adjust hormone levels accordingly without too much difficulty.

My play, *Transnormal* (2022), concerns a young man, Randall, who wants to have an operation to change into a woman. He is in love with a woman who lives in a trailer park, Patty, and whose daughter has had a sex change to become a man. Patty encourages Randall to change. His parents, Meg and Jack, are appalled at the idea. His mother says she gave birth to a son, not a daughter. His father rages against this change. The trailer park woman Patty moves on, and he has to deal with the change by himself.

Here is this play of mine:

Transnormal

Characters

Jack Bender: M, 50 years old, a transplanted New Yorker

Meg Bender: F, 45 years old, an art therapist

Randall Bender: M, 22 years old, on the spectrum

Patricia Johnson/Dr. Hughes: F, 38 years old, same actor to play Patricia and Dr. Hughes

> **Act 1, Scene 1:**
>
> An airport in Arizona. Late afternoon.
>
> **At rise:** Meg and Jack have been waiting for 2 hours. Jack is pacing. Meg is sitting.

Jack

Where is he?

Meg

He said he'd be here at 1.

Jack

It's 3. I'm so exhausted from that trip. These cruises are so draining. I just want to go home.

Meg

Take it easy, Jack. Sit down. Don't get upset.

Jack

If he pulls that no show shit with me again . . .

Meg

He'll show. Give him time.

Jack

We just gave him two hours!

Meg

Maybe there's traffic.

Jack

Let's take an Uber home.

Meg

But then when he does show up and he's searching for us . . .

Jack

Bullshit!!! You've been indulging him his whole life, which is why . . .

Meg

Please, don't fight in the airport with all these people.
(*She looks around.*)

Jack

I'm not fighting! I'm merely telling you. . . . (*looks around*)
There's no one around.

Meg

Maybe he got our flight or arrival time wrong?
(*She checks her phone.*)
I'll call again.
She calls.
(*on phone*) Hello, honey. Are you almost here? We're in the arrival lounge.

Jack

Did he answer?
(*She shakes her head no.*)
Why can't he answer his phone like a normal human being?

Meg

Don't start again with "normal" . . .

Jack

Why not? What's so weird about wanting our son to behave like a normal
human being?

Meg

Oh, Jack, please.

Jack

Let's give it a time limit. If he's not here by 3:30 . . .

Meg

Why don't you just take an Uber?

Jack

Without you?

Meg

I'll wait for him. You go home.

Jack

No, I'll wait until 3:30.

> (*Randall enters, out of breath.*)

Randall

Hi Mom! Hi Dad! Sorry to keep you waiting.

Jack

What the hell happened to you?

Meg

Stop it, Jack!

> (*She hugs Randall.*)

Randall

Patricia had the car. I had to go over to her place to get it. Then she couldn't find the keys.

Jack
(*Disgusted*)

Oh, shut up. Let's just go.

> (*He picks up two suitcases and points to Meg's suitcases for Randall to carry.*)

Meg

No, I want to hear what happened.

> (*Jack is getting angrier and angrier.
> He drops his suitcases and groans.*)

Randall

We found the keys. Then she wanted to come with me to help bring you home, but I told her that you guys do not want to see or hear from her. Isn't that right?

Jack

You bet your ass, that's right! Why are you still hanging out with that woman?

Meg

Please Jack. Lower your voice.

Jack

She's a dangerous sociopath, Randall! Can't you get that through your head? She stole my credit card, put a virus on my computer, and insulted your mother! What more does she have to do for you to get the point?

Meg

What was she doing with your car?

Randall

I let her borrow it because she had to drop her daughters off.

Meg

Which one, the one in jail?

Randall

C'mon Mom; that one has been out for months. They were all going to their grandma's.

Jack

Son, I'm trying to be tolerant, but you're driving me crazy.

Randall

I wish you could understand, Dad. Patricia is a good person if you'd only get to know her like I do.

Meg

We don't want to get to know her, dear. She's not the right kind of person for you. You'll make better friends, I'm sure.

Randall

Let me get these bags for you, Mom.

> (*He picks up Meg's bags and starts to carry them out.*)

Jack

(*Drops his bags.*)

No! I want you to promise me right here and now that you will never see that woman again!

Meg

Oh, please, not here! Not now!

> (*She's looking around.*)

Jack

Yes, here! Yes now! I want a public declaration from you, Randall! If you want to live in our house, eat our food, drive our cars, that you will NEVER see this Patricia again!

Randall

I can't do that, Dad.

Meg

Let's just go.

Jack

Why can't you do that?

Randall

She's the most important person in my life and the only one who understands me. I can't give her up.

Meg

More important than your parents?

Randall

No one's more important than you, Mom, but . . .

Meg

But what, Randall, tell us.

Randall

I love her. You know that.

Meg

But you love us too, dear. Sometimes you have to choose one person over another.

Jack

Stop with the philosophy. As you said, this is no place for any of this. We'll deal with it at home.

(*He picks up his suitcases again.*)

Randall

No one else understands me like she does. And . . . And . . .

Meg

And what, dear?

Randall

And when I have the operation, she's the only one who'll be there for me, she said.

Meg

Operation?

Jack

What operation?

(*Randall's phone rings. He stares at it, and it keeps ringing.*)

Randall

Hold on a second.

> (*He drops Meg's suitcase and answers.*)

Oh no! You're kidding? No. OK, OK. Don't worry. I'll be right there.

> (*Jack is glaring at him with disbelief, while Meg tries to stay nonchalant.*)

Sorry. Uh. I have to go. Patricia needs me. Stay here. I'll be right back.

> (*He runs out.*)

Jack

Randall!! Randall!!! Come back here! I can't believe this!

Meg

I must say it's pretty unbelievable.

Jack

He could at least lie to us. He could say: "Mom and Dad I have . . ."

Meg

You know, Jack, he doesn't have the capacity to lie.

Jack

You're right. I keep hoping against hope that he could be OK. He's got to move out. He can't stay in my house anymore.

Meg

I understand, but please remember what happened the last time you kicked him out.

Jack

Things will be different now.

Meg

In what way? He can't live on his own.

Jack
He has Patricia now. She'll take him in.

Meg
You want Patricia to take him in? Didn't you just say . . .

Jack
I know what I said. The point is I don't want him in my house anymore.

Meg
It's my house, too.

Jack
I'm getting sick from this stress. You want that? You want me to drop dead from a heart attack or something?

Meg
Take it easy, Jack. Let's get an Uber and go home.

Jack
Of course. That's what we should have done to begin with.
>   (*He takes out his phone to order a car.*)

Act 1, Scene 2: In front of Patricia's trailer. Half an hour after Scene 1.
At rise: Patricia and Randall are crouched down near her trailer.

Patricia
Thank God you got here so fast. Tortie has been stuck under there for hours. I'm afraid she'll die.

Randall
It can't be hours, Patty. I was just here an hour ago.

Patricia

You know what I mean, honey. Let's get her out.

> (*Randall squats down lower and peers under the trailer, trying to see Tortie.*)

Randall

Maybe she likes it under there and we shouldn't disturb her.

Patricia

No, she hid under there because the cat was jumping on her. Here's a piece of lettuce. Try to lure her out.

> (*Patricia takes a handful of lettuce out of her pocket and gives it to him. Randall takes it and waves it under the trailer.*)

Randall

Here boy, I mean girl. Come get some tasty lettuce.

Patricia

C'mon, Tortie, girl, c'mon out.

Randall

My parents were real mad at me.

Patricia

Aren't they always? They'll never understand.

Randall

They said I should never see you again.

Patricia

How silly of them. Did you tell them I'm a parent myself and know what they feel?

Randall

I didn't tell them that. Should I?

Patricia

Yes, with three kids of my own. I'm a mother to you all.

Randall

I can't even see Tortie under there.

Patricia

Use the light on your phone. You'll see her.

> (*Randall pulls out his phone and puts on the flashlight app.*)

Randall

She's not there.

> (*He stands up.*)

My back hurts from crouching.

Patricia

Your back shouldn't hurt at your age.

> (*She stands up, too.*)

Randall

Let's look for her somewhere else.

> (*Patricia laughs.*)

Patricia

I saw her crawl under there. That's where she has to be. You know a turtle can't move that fast.

Randall

She could have crawled out the back. My father also said you stole his credit card, put a virus on his computer, and insulted my mother.

Patricia

He said all that about me? First of all, I only borrowed his credit card with your permission. Second, that virus came on because he didn't have an antivirus thingamajig on his computer. And how in the world did I insult your mother?

Randall

Didn't you say my mother was a phony or something like that?

Patricia

I was just saying what I felt. She's not the most genuine woman I ever met.

Randall

Anyway, what should I do if they don't want me to see you?

Patricia

Do you want to see me?

Randall

Yes, you are my lifesaver.

Patricia

Thank you, honey. I feel the same. They can't stop us. You are 22 and legal.

Randall

They don't want me in their house.

Patricia

Well, you can stay with us, but it will be a little crowded.

Randall

I can sleep outdoors here in your hammock.

Patricia

You stay with them as long as you can. If you do get kicked out, we'll deal with it.

Randall

Thank you. You're always so helpful.

Patricia

Let's sit out here in case Tortie comes out. Want me to do your horoscope today?

> (*They sit down in two folding chairs in front of the trailer.*)

Randall

Yes, please.

Patricia
(*Looking up at the sky.*)
Today the moon is in Sagittarius, the sun is in Virgo, Mercury is retrograde. So let's see, since you're a Virgo you might have difficult people like your parents bothering you, but you can rest assured you'll come out ahead of the game with them.

Randall

That's so accurate. And that time you did my chart it was amazing.

Patricia

I think I just have a natural flare for astrology. I don't have to do much to get it right.

Randall

The best part was when you told me I was supposed to be a woman and something went wrong.

Patricia

I know you liked that. You feel like a woman deep inside, don't you Randy?

Randall

Yes, that's how I feel. My parents told me I was ridiculous for feeling like that, and I would get over it.

Patricia

I'm sure they meant well.

Randall

I don't think my father means well. He hates me.

Patricia

Maybe he hates himself. I think it's time we look for Tortie again, Randy.
                                    (*Randall crouches down and
                                    looks under the trailer again,*

shining his iPhone light under there.)

Not there?

Randall

I don't see her.

Patricia

Give me your phone.

(She scrolls through his phone.)

You know what, now that the kids are at Grandma's for a while, we can do some microdosing.

Randall

Are you sure that's OK?

Patricia

Sure. The stars and moon are aligned just right for it. I wouldn't lead you astray.

Randall

Last time we took . . .

Patricia

That was a full dose. Now this here (she pulls out a plastic bag full of pills) is just a teeny tiny dose. No harm will befall us.

(She surreptitiously puts some in her mouth.)

Randall

I better prepare myself.

(He takes some deep breaths and looks anxious.)

Patricia

I put a little in Tortie's food, too. Sort of like an experiment to see what would happen.

Randall

Maybe that's why she's hiding.

Patricia

You sure are one smart boy. I don't know why they said you are . . . you know.

Randall

I am very good at math and chess, and I remember everything.

Patricia

I love you, baby.

> (*They kiss and give each other a big hug.*)

Randall

> (*Trying to spit something out of his mouth.*)

Ugh, something got into my mouth.

Patricia

Don't spit it out! It's the microdose. Here wash it down.

> (*She hands him a can of diet soda. He swallows it.*)

Randall

How long will it take . . .

Patricia

Not long! Let's dance.

> (*She puts on some music (Meatloaf or equivalent)*)
> (*They dance when—*)

Jack
(*Enters in a huff.*)

There you are!

Meg
(*Enters not far behind.*)
I told you to take it easy, Jack.

Patricia
Welcome to my humble abode. Let me get you . . .

Jack
Don't bother. This is not a social visit. Randall, come here!

> (*Randall goes over to his mother and holds her hand. They smile at each other.*)

Randall
Hi, Dad.

Jack
I want you to leave my son alone, or I'll get an order of protection from the court.

Patricia
Now, now, Mr. Bender. Let's not get all excited, like your wife says.

Jack
Ever since you started seeing him, he's been worse than ever.

Patricia
Worse in what way? He seems better to me.

Meg
We don't think so.

> (*Randall is smiling broadly, and he keeps hugging his mother.*)

Stop it, Randall. Not now.

Patricia
Really? Look how friendly he is. I don't suppose he was hugging and kissing you before.

Meg

He wasn't. Randall has always been averse to touching since he was a baby. I don't know what's gotten into him.

Patricia

Well, look at him now. Friendly as a little puppy.

Jack

That's probably a bad sign for a boy on the spectrum. Maybe he's having a breakdown.

Patricia

(*Laughing.*)

You both are so wrapped up in what your experts told you long ago that you can't see what's in front of your eyes right now. He's fine.

Jack

Stop it! How dare you, an uneducated piece of, piece of . . . trash, tell us what's good for our son!

Meg

Please Jack! There's no need for insults and shouting. You're scaring Randall. Let's just get out of here. Come, son. We're going.

> (*Randall is cringing as Jack yells and carries on.*)

Jack

I'll say when it's time to go. I want to have this out with her.

Patricia

There's nothing to have out. If your son feels like going with you, he will. You can't force people.

Jack

You should talk! You're forcing him or somehow coercing him to be with you. I want you to stop it.

Patricia
(*To Randall.*)
Am I forcing you to be with me?

Randall
No, I want to be here.

Patricia
See?

Meg
Randall, please come with us.
> (*She looks pleadingly into his eyes.*)

Randall
OK, Mom.
> (*He is holding his mother's hand and they exit.*)

Patricia
Talk about forcing. I think you two are doing that to him. But you'll see.
> (*Jack comes very close to Patricia with his hand raised. She doesn't flinch.*)

Jack
I want to smack you, but I won't because . . .

Patricia
You won't, Mister, and you can bet I'll sue you but good, if you do.
> (*She laughs and Jack exits in a huff.*)

Act 1, Scene 3: The next night in Meg's bedroom.
At rise: Meg is sitting on her bed looking unhappy. A knock on the door.

Randall
(Calling from Off Stage)

May I come in, Mom?

Meg

Of course, dear. Sit right here.

> *(Randall enters. Meg pats the spot next to her on the bed, and Randall sits there.)*

Randall

Patricia says I have to talk to you.

Meg

You can always talk to me. You certainly don't need her permission.

Randall

I guess so.

Meg

Have you been feeling OK? Still getting those headaches?

Randall

I'm feeling better. I want to tell you . . .

Meg

I understand—Patricia is your lover, and you want to tell me?

Randall

Yes, but . . .

Meg

She is so much older than you. And she has three children.

Randall

Mary Ann, Nedi, and Gabby.

Meg

You like them?

Randall

They're all great. I love the whole family, Mom.

Meg

What about the father?

Randall

Who knows? They all have different fathers, I think. We don't talk about them.

Meg

I suppose you want to be the father of another one?

Randall

It's not that, Mom.

Meg

I always pictured you with a woman your own age.

Randall

Patricia is only 38!

Meg

So that's what, sixteen years your senior.

Randall

I don't want to talk about that.

Meg

Then what is it, dear?

Randall

Well, it is about sex.

Meg

I don't feel comfortable hearing about your sex life with her.

Randall

We do it, but Patricia likes girls better.

Meg

Oh, is that right? Then what is she doing with . . .

Randall

Well, she's with me now, but I will, I . . . , I . . .

Meg
(*Turns and stares at him.*)
What? What are you saying?

Randall

I'm going to . . . Mom, have you noticed my breasts?
(*He sticks his chest out.*)

Meg
(*Looking at his chest.*)
I saw that, dear, but I thought you were gaining a little weight or smoking marijuana perhaps?

Randall

No, Mom. It's hormones.

Meg

Oh no! You can't mean. . . . Is that why you said an operation? Is that what you're going to have, a sex change operation?

Randall

Yes, Mom.

Meg
(*Crying.*)
No! You can't mean that! I can't condone that.
(*She hugs him desperately.*)
You're my little boy! I had a little baby boy, not a girl.
(*She's crying. They're hugging.*)

Randall

I've been meaning to tell you.

Meg

It's impossible! Whatever you do, don't tell your father!

Randall

No, I'm just telling you.

Meg

You're way past puberty, so won't the hormones be harmful?

Randall

No, the doctors say it's no problem. I feel better with them.

Meg

Are you doing it for her? So you can become her lesbian lover?

Randall

Don't be mad, Mom. If I can't have the operation, I might . . .

Meg

It's illegal, isn't it? In Arizona?

Randall

Not at all. I go to a clinic where I see a therapist just for this. He thinks I'm fine. They have the doctors there all ready when I am.

Meg

And you didn't tell me until now! Don't you trust me, Randall?

Randall

I knew you wouldn't like it.

Meg

Did Patricia encourage this?

Randall

She's very supportive. Her daughter, Gabby, was a boy, and she had the operation.

Meg

But it's different for you. You are a disabled person, Randall. You can't make these kind of decisions for yourself. I'm sure you'll need parental approval.

Randall

I don't feel disabled. When I'm with Patricia I feel so able.

Meg

I won't allow it!

> (*She's crying and holding on to Randall.*)

You're my baby boy.

Randall

Ah, Mom, I know. You feel bad, but I need this for my life, for my . . .

Meg

You don't have the money. I'm sure it costs a fortune.

Randall

I've been saving.

Meg

I thought you were giving all your money to that woman.

Randall

She's saving it for me.

Meg

That's ridiculous! What little you earn, you must keep for yourself, but not for an operation.

Randall

Patricia is keeping my money in a special account just for this.

Meg

You're kidding? You can't trust her. She's a sociopath.

Jack
(*Entering.*)
I'm so tired. I just want to go to sleep. Oh, hi, Randall. So nice to see you here and talking to your mother.

> (*They both stare at him guiltily.*)

Act 1, Scene 4: The next morning.
At rise: Randall is banging furiously at Patricia's trailer door.

Randall

Patricia!! Patricia!!

Patricia
(*Peeks out her door.*)
What is it? Oh hi, Randy. It's too early in the morning for us.

Randall

I told my mother.

Patricia

Very good, Randy! Let me get my coffee and come out.
> (*She shuts the door. Randall looks under the trailer and all around. She comes back out with two cups of coffee and hands one to Randall.*)

Randall

Thank you.

Patricia
(*Yawning.*)
Sit down and tell me all about it.

Randall

She didn't like it. She wants me to talk to a surgeon friend of hers who'll explain what the surgery will be like.

Patricia

I wouldn't do that if I were you. It'll just scare you.

Randall

I'm worried she'll tell my father, and then he'll stop it. I made her promise not to.

Patricia

Listen, honey, as long as you're here, I have something important to tell you.

Randall

What?

Patricia

A new company bought this property, and they doubled the rent on my lot. I'm going to need a lot more money.

Randall

You need more money? I'll work two shifts, I mean . . .

Patricia

It won't be enough. I know we can't ask your parents for it.

Randall

No way. We already used Dad's credit card to buy these chairs and . . .

Patricia

Yeah, and he was so pissed.

Randall

Let's sell something or could you park somewhere else?

Patricia

I've got to park in a RV lot or I'll get towed. That happened one time . . .

Randall

I need you to be here.

Patricia

You're going to do this on your own. I got you connected to that clinic. Just keep going there. They'll take care of you.

Randall

I can't face my parents without you.

Patricia

Yes, you can, baby. I have to go back to California. My mother took my kids, and she's threatening me.

Randall

What's she doing?

Patricia

She said if I don't go back to L.A. and live in an apartment like a normal person, she's going to take my kids from me.

Randall

You don't want to go to L.A.

Patricia

I'm glad I got out of there, but she's forcing me to go back. She's kind of like your father.

Randall

Why do people interfere so much with us?

Patricia

That's just how they are.

Randall

Please, please, stay, Patricia. You know my life is worth nothing without you.

Patricia

You are so sweet, and I can't wait to see you as a woman.

(*She kisses and hugs him.*)

Randall

I won't have the strength to do it without you.

Patricia

Of course you will. I'll come back and be with you after.

Randall

(*Gets down on one knee.*)

OK. I've been wanting to . . . Will you marry me, Patricia?

Patricia

(*Laughing.*)

You got a ring? Oh, get up, silly. That won't make me stay.

Randall

(*Gets up.*)

What will make you stay?

Patricia

Maybe if you were a millionaire? Or if you could provide me and my kids with a big beautiful house. Or . . .

Randall

You know I can't do any of that. Is there something I can do?

Act 1, Scene 5: That evening Meg and Jack are at home, relaxing after their exhausting cruise. **At rise:** Meg is in the kitchen unpacking groceries.

Jack

I'm so glad to be home. Let's relax with a nice dinner, just the three of us.

Meg

I went shopping and bought everything for tacos. I can make them with gua-camole, jack cheese, and refried beans.

> (*While she unpacks the groceries, Jack looks out the window.*)

Jack

Hey, isn't that your friend, what's his name, the surgeon. He's talking to Randall?

Meg

Yes. It's Dr. Jason. I asked him to stop by and talk to him.

Jack

What for?

Meg

Remember Randall mentioned an operation when we were at the airport?

Jack

Yeah, I thought that was strange. Did you find out why?

Meg

OK, Jack. Please sit down for this one.

> (*He reluctantly sits down.*)

Meg

Dr. Jason, Jim, is now specializing in sex reassignment surgery.

Jack

Oh, shit!!! No!!! You mean . . .

Meg

Yeah, Jack.

> (*Jack stands up.*)

No, sit down, sit down.

Jack

Oh, no! It can't. . . . He won't!!! I won't let him!

Meg

That's exactly what I said.

Jack

Fuck no!!! On top of everything he wants to do that! I thought he was in love with a woman? How can he want to . . . He wants to get castrated? He's crazy!!

Meg

So I figured if he talked to Jim and understood what it really meant to have that surgery.

Jack

Brilliant! That's a brilliant idea! People don't understand what real surgery involves. I know when I had my knee operation how hard that was. And it took so long to recuperate.

Meg

Exactly, so I hope Randall will change his mind when he hears the facts.

Jack
(*Kisses her.*)

My clever Meg.

Meg
(*Kisses him back.*)

And I have good news for you too! Patricia is leaving Arizona!! She has to go back to L.A.

Jack

Hooray!!! That is the best news I've heard for weeks! We have to celebrate!!!

Meg

Yes, that's the best thing that could happen.

Jack

And once Patricia is gone, he'll be out from under her bad influence. I bet she set him up for the operation. We can convince him otherwise.

Meg

We have to convince him. I think we can do it. You know he's taking hormones already.

Jack

I noticed that he seemed to have breasts, but I was ignoring it.

Meg

I was, too. I thought that woman was making him smoke marijuana.

Jack

I'm so glad she's going!! Now we'll be able to get him to come to his senses.

> (*Randall runs in, all upset and dashes past them into his room.*)

Jack
(*Cont.*)

Randall!!! Randall!! Buddy, speak to me.

Meg

Leave him alone for now. Jim must have upset him.

> (*They both look out the window.*)

Meg
(*Cont.*)

He's driving off. Jim said he had an appointment and would just stop by for a few minutes to talk to Randall. I'll call him later.

Jack

Let Randall cool down. We'll talk at dinner. I'll make a salad to go with the tacos. That's what was missing on the cruise, enough veggies to round out the meals.

Meg

They're always skimpy on the veggies. Next year I want to take another cruise.

Jack

Whoa! Wait a minute. We just got home. What about my work? I don't want my business to go down the tubes.

Meg

You know you can be like a workaholic sometimes.

Jack

That's not fair. I've supported you and Randall all these years because I work hard. If I leave my business unsupervised, these workers play around.

Meg

I know, Jack, but we've got to enjoy our lives, too.

Jack

I enjoy my work. Anyway, we were just gone for 18 days, so I don't want to go anywhere any time soon. I'm just glad to be home.

Meg

I am, too. And we're back just in time to help Randall.

Jack

Yes, imagine if when we came home, he'd already had the surgery and . . .

Meg

What a nightmare that would have been.

Jack

Where would he get the money anyway?

Meg

Patricia certainly couldn't have provided it.

Jack

No way! She was trying to rip us off.

Meg

She did rip us off!! And took the little money he made.

> (*There's a loud thud. They look at each other.*)

Jack

What was that? Let me go see.

(*He exits. Meg calls after him.*)

Meg
(*Yelling.*)
Be nice, Jack! Tell him we're having tacos for dinner. He loves them.

Jack
(*O. S., knocking on a door.*)
Randall!!! Randall!! Come out, son!! We're going to have tacos! Your favorite. (*A few beats.*)

Randall!! Randall!!! I'm coming in. (*A few beats.*)

Oh my God!!! No!!! No!!! It can't be!!!

Meg
(*Exits; we hear her from O. S.*)
NO!!!! I can't believe it!!!

(*She screams.*)

Jack
(*O. S.*)
Call 911!!! NOW!!!! Fast! I'll cut him down!!

Act 2, Scene 1: On the ward of a psychiatric hospital, in the office of Dr. Hughes, a psychiatrist. Meg and Jack are waiting for the doctor and Randall.

Jack

I hate this place. Last time he was in, I . . .

Meg

Well, I don't like it any better than you. But whatever you do, don't go yelling at the doctor again.

Jack

The last one who treated him was a complete idiot. I didn't mean to yell at him, but he was so ridiculous. And apparently he didn't help Randall, if he wound up in here again.

Meg

We've got to help Randall any way we can. So if he has to be here, OK. Let him get straightened out.

Jack

I don't think he'll ever get straightened out with his condition.

Dr. Hughes
(*Enters.*)

Hello, Mr. and Ms. Bender. I'm so glad to meet you. Thanks for coming in.
                                        (*She shakes both their hands and
                                        takes a seat behind her desk.*)

Meg

How is Randall?

Dr. Hughes

He's much better. He'll be joining us momentarily. He's just getting his meds.

Jack

What are you giving him?

Dr. Hughes

Just some tranquilizers to keep him calm. He was quite upset about losing his girlfriend.

Meg

Did he tell you about her?

Dr. Hughes

He did. Would you like to add anything?

Jack

Did he tell you she's 38 with three kids?

Dr. Hughes

Yes, he said he enjoyed being with her and the whole family. It was quite a shock to him when she left.

Meg

Did he happen to mention that she convinced him to have a sex change operation?

Dr. Hughes

He didn't say that she convinced him. He said he wanted that since before puberty, but he was too timid to tell you about it.

Jack

Bullshit! That sociopath talked him into it because she's a lesbian and wanted him to be her female lover.

Dr. Hughes

Interesting theory. Randall would be the type to be persuaded more easily than other people, but he seems to want the sex change anyway.

Meg

Do you recommend that for him?

Dr. Hughes

It's not for us to recommend it, but if patients want that we don't dissuade them.

Jack

Why not? It's crazy for a boy like that to destroy his body.

Dr. Hughes

But look what happened when your surgeon friend described the gory details to Randall. And this was not the first time he tried to kill himself.

Meg

Are you blaming us for that?

Dr. Hughes

I'm not blaming anyone. I'm just pointing out that Randall has his mind made up.

Meg

He was going to some clinic where he was seeing a therapist, and they were getting him ready for the operation.

Dr. Hughes

Yes, he told me about that.

Jack

And? Is it a reputable place? What kind of therapist would recommend that?

Dr. Hughes

I never heard of it. I'll have to do some research and find out about it.

Jack

I'm sure it's a sleazy place that just sucks the money out of people for these operations.

Randall
(*Enters.*)

Hi Mom, Dad. Good to see you.

> (*Dr. Hughes points to a seat, and Randall sits down.*)

Meg

How are you feeling?

Randall

Better, Mom.

> (*Jack reaches over and gives Randall a hug.*)

Jack
So glad to hear that, son.

Meg
How long do you think Randall will be in here?

Dr. Hughes
Randall, are you still feeling like hurting yourself?
> (*Randall nods yes and keeps his head down.*)

Jack
But why, Randall? You have everything a person could want. A good home, two devoted parents, all the food you can eat; we'll take you wherever you want and do practically anything for you.

Randall
I don't have Patricia, and I'm a guy.

Meg
Is that what it is?

Dr. Hughes
It just goes to show you that a person can have every material thing he or she could desire, be beautiful or handsome, and still want to commit suicide. I've seen it too many times. Look at all these celebrities who want to kill themselves. People think they have everything.

Meg
Randall is not a celebrity, but as Jack said we gave him everything we could.

Jack
Do you think we spoiled him?

Meg
Maybe we shouldn't talk about him in front of him like this. What do you think, doctor?

Dr. Hughes

No. It's better not to have secrets and talk behind his back. Is it OK with you that we are talking like this?

Randall

Yes. I want to hear this.

Meg

I ask myself, what did I do wrong? I'd do anything for my son, but I don't want him to turn into a girl.

Dr. Hughes

What if you ask yourself, why not? What would be the harm if he became your daughter?

Jack

That's ridiculous! We have a son. Why would we want him to be anything but?

Meg
(*Crying.*)

Before Randall was born, I had three terrible miscarriages and one still birth, who they told me was a girl. When I finally gave birth to my little baby boy, I was so happy to have him. He was so adorable. Then when they told me he was autistic, I . . . I . . .

> (*Jack hugs her. Randall looks upset.*)

Dr. Hughes

I understand. Take your time, Ms. Bender.

> (*She offers Meg a tissue.*)

Randall

Maybe that was me. The stillbirth girl. I was trying to come into this world and . . .

Jack

What are you talking about, Randall! Can't you see your mother is upset?

> (*Randall hangs his head.*)

Dr. Hughes

It's better not to be so harsh and dismissive with Randall. He's a sensitive person.

Jack

Well, I can't stand it when he talks nonsense.

Dr. Hughes

It's not nonsense to him. He's trying to express himself the best he can.

Meg

You're right of course. He has to express himself, but we feel so terrible about this.

Jack

Dr. Hughes, I want to ask you. Why are there so many cases of boys turning into girls and girls turning into boys? This can't be normal.

Dr. Hughes

In psychiatry we used to believe this was abnormal. In fact, homosexuality was considered abnormal and a mental illness up until 1973, when our diagnostic manual reclassified it as a variation on normal. Now what Randall has is called gender dysphoria. In other words, he is dissatisfied with his present sex. I think the world and the people in it are changing rapidly, and we have to adapt to it.

Jack
(*Yelling.*)

That's absurd! I don't give a good goddamn what you call it! It's abnormal to me and most of society!

> (*Meg puts her hand on Jack's arm to calm him. He shrugs her off.*)

Stop it, Meg!

Meg

Sorry, doctor. Jack yells like that when he gets excited.

Dr. Hughes

It's OK. I can understand that this is upsetting him. However, you know Randall has started the sex change process by taking female hormones.

Meg

Did you continue to give him those hormones?

Dr. Hughes

We did. He would feel even worse if we stopped them abruptly.

Jack

Come on, you have to stop them! We'll deal with whatever happens.

Dr. Hughes

No. Randall is getting what we call "gender-affirming" care on this ward. We think that's the best plan for him.

> (*Jack stands up and is shouting. Randall cowers as he does that.*)

Jack

I want him out of here at once! I'll take him home or . . . or

Meg

(*Grabbing his arm.*)

Sit down, dear. Do you think all this yelling had a bad effect on Randall in his childhood?

> (*Jack sits down and glares at the doctor. He is attempting to quiet himself.*)

Dr. Hughes

Remember we're not blaming anyone. I'm just asking that we respect each other's opinions no matter how strange they may seem. As long as I have you both here, I'd like to ask you some questions, if I may?

Meg

What do you want to know?

Dr. Hughes

When was Randall first diagnosed with autism?

Jack

(*In control and trying to cooperate.*)

Wasn't he about four?

Meg

No, it was earlier—at two. I always think I must have eaten too many processed meats or swallowed toxins in my food or was I breathing polluted air?

Dr. Hughes

Ms. Bender, we think autism is a complex neurodevelopmental disorder. Don't think it was your fault. We're not sure what causes it. It could be genetics mixed with certain environmental pollutants. Many studies have been done, but they're all inconclusive.

Meg

(*Upset.*)

I've always blamed myself.

Jack

And I've always told her not to. We love him no matter what.

Randall

If you love me, please accept me.

Meg

We are trying to. Please understand that, Randall. That's why we're here.

Dr. Hughes

It will take them some time, Randall. This is not easy for people of their generation to understand.

Meg

Do you think it's easier for people of his generation to understand this?

Dr. Hughes

Yes, I think so.

Act 2, Scene 3: The morning after scene 2. In the Bender's kitchen. They've just had news that Randall escaped the ward.
At rise: Meg is getting ready to leave.

Meg

Hurry up, Jack!!! Where are you? We have to go find him!

Jack
(*Enters.*)

What did the doctor say exactly?

Meg

She said that Randall was missing when they did the patient count this morning.

Jack

How could those idiots let him escape when they know he's suicidal? It's a locked ward, for God's sake!

Meg

It's not a prison. They only have one guard who sits at the door. Maybe he went to the bathroom, and Randall slipped out. Dr. Hughes said it happens all the time.

Jack

If they know it happens all the time, they should have found a way to prevent people from escaping.

Meg

Come on! We'll find him. He's probably on foot. How far could he get?

Jack

Did they look everywhere in the hospital?

Meg

She said they did. And they alerted the police.

Jack

I'm really feeling bad about this. He's suicidal.

Meg

Let's go!

Jack

Where? Maybe he went back to the RV lot where that woman was.

Meg

That doesn't make sense.

Jack

You never know with him. He doesn't always make sense. He's so sentimental. He probably wants to kiss the ground she walked on.

(*They exit. A few beats and . . .*)

Randall
(*Enters.*)

At least I found you, girl.

(*He places the turtle in the sink, opens the refrigerator, takes out some juice and drinks it straight from the container. Then he dials the landline. Speaking on the phone.*)

Hello, this is Randall. May I speak to Patricia?

(*A few beats.*)

Hi, Patty!!! I'm fine!! How is L.A.?

Well, I don't like it here either. I found Tortie. She was in the bushes behind the lot. When can I see you? You have to come back. I tried to hitchhike to L.A. but nobody would pick me up.

Phone sex? No way! I can't, Patricia. I don't think I can ever touch myself again.

No! No!! My roommate in the hospital cut off his willie. Yeah, you know, his willie! Horrible!! Blood all over the floor and bed, and he passed out. They rushed in to get him, and I rushed out of there.

I was in there because.... Never mind. I was in there. I don't know why he did it. Oh, maybe I do.

No! No!! I would never do that.

Dr. Jason said that's what they do when they give you the sex change operation. They cut it off. I don't think I can take that.

I miss you so much. I figured out that I am you and you are me and . . .

Yes, just like the song.

Wait! Wait a second!

> (*He is gagging and retching. He puts the phone down, takes Tortie out of the sink and throws up there. Then he picks up the phone again.*)

I had to throw up. Hello? Hello, Patricia? Are you still there?

> (*He hangs up reluctantly and washes out the sink. Meg rushes back in.*)

Meg
(*Enters.*)
Where is my . . . ? Randall, my baby, my boy!! You're here!! We were about to go look for you, but I forgot my phone.

Randall
Hi, Mom.

> (*They hug.*)

Meg
Are you all right? I was so upset when I heard you left the hospital. How smart of you to come back here.

Randall

I'm OK. I couldn't stay in there a minute longer.

Meg

I totally understand. Who would want to be in that horrible place?

> (*She yells out the window.*)

Meg
(*Cont.*)

Jack!!! Jack!!! Come in here!!

> (*She and Randall are hugging and crying.*)

Randall

Don't cry, Mom. I'm OK; really I am.

Jack
(*Enters.*)

What is it? Oh, Randall!! My boy!!

> (*He joins them in a group hug. They're all crying.*)

I'm so glad to see you!!! Of course you're here.

Meg

Let's all sit down and talk like civilized people.

> (*They all sit down.*)

Jack

I wanted you out of that hospital, too. Were they terrible to you there?

Randall

No. Everyone was nice.

Jack

We'll get you some good treatment. Don't worry.

Meg

But you must promise us never to try that again.

Randall

I don't think I can promise that.

Jack

You mean you would try to hang or kill yourself again?

(*Randall hangs his head.*)

Jack

(*Continued*)

Randall, look at me son. We love you too much to lose you. You're everything we want. I mean . . .

Randall

You want me as a son, and I can't be that.

Meg

I'll learn to take you any way you want to be, Randall. I want that.

Randall

Really, Mom? Ever since I was little, I felt I was in the wrong body. When I was with Patricia, I felt her body was what I wanted.

Jack

You wanted her body, or you . . . ?

Randall

I wanted to be in her body. To be her, I guess.

Jack

That is weird, son.

Meg

Don't say that, Jack. He's trying to express himself. Remember what Dr. Hughes said.

Jack

I know what she said. I have to express myself, too.

Meg

But that's the problem. We have been expressing ourselves to the exclusion of giving Randall a chance to express himself. I understand that now.

Randall

I think so.

Jack

Well, let's make a deal. Could we do that, son? Remember how we used to play that game where I'd give you a Hershey bar if you could spell all the words forward and backward in your reader?

Randall

Yes.

Jack

OK. Here's the deal: You promise not to try to kill yourself, and I'll buy you whatever you want. Not over $5,000 though.

Meg

His life is only worth $5,000 to you?

Jack

Of course not. I'm just trying to reach a compromise. You understand that, Randall, don't you?

Randall

I want a ticket to L.A.

Jack

What's in L.A.?

Meg

Patricia! You can't negotiate a business deal with something like this, Jack.

Jack

Why the hell not? But don't ask for a ticket to L.A., please. ·

> (*They hear a car stop in front of their house. Meg looks out the window.*)

Meg
It's the police. They must be looking for Randall.

Jack
(*To Randall.*)

Quick. Go hide in your room!

> (*Randall runs out to hide in his room. There's loud knocking. Jack exits to answer it.*)

Jack
(*O. S.*)

What's up? Did you find my son?

Voice
(*O. S.*)

No, sir. We thought he might have returned home. You know many escaped mental patients return to where they live.

Jack
(*O. S.*)

That makes sense. We'll be on the lookout for him if he shows up here.

Voice
(*O. S.*)

OK., thanks. Let's go, Jose.

Jack
(*Enters.*)

That was a close call.

Meg
(*Whispering.*)

You don't think we should send him back to the hospital? What if he tries that again?

Jack
I'll protect him. I'll talk to him. I'll do everything to keep him safe this time. You'll see.

Meg

Oh, Jack.

(*They hug and cry.*)

I couldn't take it if he tries it again.

Act 2: Scene 3: A few minutes after scene 2.
At rise: Jack and Randall are having a tête-à-
tête in Randall's bedroom.

Randall

Thanks, Dad, for not turning me in.

Jack

We have a deal, son. As long as I know you won't hurt yourself.

(*Randall hangs his head. A few
beats and . . .*)

Randall

OK.

Jack

It's a deal?

Randall

Yes.

(*Jack hugs Randall.*)

Jack

I'm so glad. Please explain yourself. What's going on? Do you really want to be a woman? My guess is that you admire your mother so much.

Randall

Yes, and Patricia. I know you don't like her but I do.

Jack

I don't know. Maybe she has some redeeming qualities that I missed.

Randall

You don't really know her.

Jack

I guess not, but she's in L.A., so we don't have to worry about her anymore.

Randall

I want to see her.

Jack

Maybe we can get a nice girlfriend for you, around your age.

Randall

I don't know.

Jack

What about where you work, at Amazon? Isn't there anybody there?

Randall

No.

Jack

You like girls, don't you?

Randall

I like Patricia.

Jack

What was so special about her?

Randall

She loved me.

Jack

Ah, son. What's not to love? . . . You are the cutest, sweetest person. We all love you.

Randall

Not like that.

Jack

Are you talking about sex or love or?

Randall

Both.

Jack

I'm confused. Love, I think I understand, but . . . Well, let me just say . . .

Randall

Please, Dad.

> (*He hangs his head and covers his ears.*)

Jack

I'm embarrassing you?

Randall

Yes.

Jack

What did you do with Patricia, may I ask?

Randall

No, Dad.

> (*Randall interrupts himself with giggling.*)

Jack

I blame myself, you know. When I was teaching you about sex maybe I concentrated on the safe sex, condom part, too much. I should have given you a better sex education, but I wanted you to be safe.

Randall

This is weird, when you talk like this.

Jack

I'm just trying to know you better, son. That's weird?

> (*Randall nods.*)

Randall

I want to go.

Jack

Where? You're home, safe and sound.

Randall

L.A.

Jack

Impossible! If you want me to start yelling again, just keep this up. You're not going to L.A.

Randall

Dad, you said we have a deal. Help me.

Jack

I'm trying, son, but you have to be reasonable. You just got out of the hospital. You're not ready to travel so far.

Randall

382.2 miles is not so far.

Jack

It certainly is. I would say that drive would take us about eight hours or more.

Randall

I want to go.

Jack

NO! Stop it. Let's talk about something else. You know I always thought we'd do everything together. Father and son stuff. I'd take you with me wherever I went. When you were seven you followed me around all the time. We'd play chess, and you always won. I got such a kick out of that. Your little hand clutching your queen. Your beautiful face tight with concentration. I could watch you forever.

Randall

I want to go or no deal.

Jack

What do you mean no deal?

(*The police have returned and are questioning Meg.*)

Meg
(*O. S.*)

Jack, may I speak with you for a minute?

Jack

OK. I'll be right there.

(*He exits. We hear people speaking in the next room, but we can't hear the words.*)

Randall
(*To himself.*)

No deal. No deal.

Jack
(*Enters.*)

Do we have a deal or not?

Randall

Are we going to L.A.?

Jack

Absolutely not.

Randall

Then no deal.

Meg
(*Enters.*)

Can they come in now?

Jack

Pack your things, son.

Randall

NO! NO! NO!

> (*Randall tries to hide under the bed. Jack grabs him and tries to hold him, but he escapes and runs out into the kitchen, where the cops have returned to take him back to the hospital. Meg called them.*)

Randall
(O. S.)

NO! No, No, leave me alone! I won't go. Stop it.

Jack
(*To Meg.*)

I hope they won't hurt him.

Meg

It would be worse if we left him here and he hurt himself.

Act 2: Scene 3: Back in the psychiatric hospital. This time in the "quiet room," a padded room. At rise: Randall is curled into a ball and rocking.

Dr. Hughes
(*Enters.*)

Hello, Randall.

> (*No response from Randall.*)

How are you today?

> (*No response.*)

Sorry that you have to be in here.

> (*No response.*)

I heard that you haven't eaten for three days.

Randall
(*Mumbling.*)

Two.

Dr. Hughes

I can't hear you, and I so want to. Can you sit back and say that again, please.

Randall
(*Sitting up.*)

Two days!

Dr. Hughes

Thank you for answering! I stand corrected. Two days.

Randall

Not hungry.

Dr. Hughes

If you go too many days without food, I'll have to transfer you to a medical floor. There they'll put a tube down your throat into your stomach and feed you. You don't want that, do you?

Randall

No.

Dr. Hughes

I know the food is terrible here, but you have to try to eat. Would you like me to ask your parents to bring you something better?

Randall
(*Shakes his head no.*)

I want to go.

Dr. Hughes

You mean go out of the quiet room to the regular part of the ward?

Randall

No, home.

Dr. Hughes

Do you think you're ready to go home?

Randall

Yes.

Dr. Hughes

The way it works is this: You eat first, then you go back to the regular ward. When you're not suicidal anymore, you can go home.

Randall

How do I get not suicidal?

Dr. Hughes

You talk to me, take your meds, and attend groups.

Randall

I can talk to you.

Dr. Hughes

Great. I'm glad you feel that way. I brought you something.

> (*She takes a chess set out of her bag and sets it up on the floor where they are both sitting.*)

Randall

(*Looks interested.*)

No one wants to play with me anymore.

Dr. Hughes

That's because you are so good! Your parents said you beat everyone every time.

Randall

I play against the computer.

> (*Dr. Hughes takes a white piece and a black piece, holds one in each hand behind her back, and*

> *then she holds both closed fists in front of her for Randall to choose. He taps her right fist.)*

> *(She opens her fist. He has chosen the black one. They set the pieces on the board and begin to play.)*

This one.

Dr. Hughes

I used to play in college, but like you said not many people want to play anymore.

Randall

(*Moves a piece.*)
I'm fast, too.

Dr. Hughes

(*Studying the board.*)
I'll just get my knight out here.

Randall

No! No! Bad move.
(*He leans forward and makes a great move.*)

Dr. Hughes

Oh, I see what you mean.

Randall

You should have seen it first and played Queen's pawn opening.
(*He points to the pieces.*)

Dr. Hughes

You'll have to teach me that and more.

Randall
(*Making moves.*)
I'm class A. I only need a few more points to be an Expert. Now watch this!
>(*There's a knock on the door and an off-stage voice.*)

Attendant
(*O. S.*)
His lunch is here, doctor.

Dr. Hughes
(*Makes a move and then gets up.*)
I'll take it.
>(She takes a tray from him and sets it down next to Randall.)

Randall
You are in trouble.
>(*He shoves the tray away from him and makes a move.*)

Dr. Hughes
(*Examining the tray.*)
You want this? Or how about this?
>(*She takes a peanut butter and jelly sandwich out of her bag and shows it to Randall.*)

Randall
(*Makes a move.*)
After this.

Dr. Hughes
(*Setting the sandwich near him.*)
OK. Let me see. I think I'll move here.

Randall

Terrible move!! Watch!!

> (*He moves his pieces quickly and dazzles Dr. Hughes.*)

CHECKMATE!!!

Dr. Hughes

Oh, no!! You're just too good. That was amazing! Do you feel . . .

> (*Randall grabs the sandwich.*)

Randall

Yes!

> (*He rips off the saran wrap and devours the sandwich.*)

My fave!

Dr. Hughes

Slowly please. You haven't eaten in two days. When you break a fast you must eat very slowly and carefully.

> (*She pours a glass of water for him from the tray. He starts choking and coughing.*)

Dr. Hughes
(*Cont.*)

May I pat you on the back?

Randall
(*Coughing.*)

Yes.

> (*She pats him on the back and then hands him the water, which he drinks.*)

Dr. Hughes

Very good, Randall. Let me see you eat for two more days, and then you'll go to the regular ward.

Randall
(*Collecting himself.*)
I don't want to go to the regular ward.

Dr. Hughes
Remember that's how you advance to going home.

Randall
I had a roommate. . . .

Dr. Hughes
Oh yes. Your roommate. That must have been so frightening for you.

Randall
He cut off his . . .

Dr. Hughes
I know it was horrible, especially for you.

Randall
Where did he go?

Dr. Hughes
He went to surgery. I think they were able to reattach it. He'll be back here when he's better. Right now he's not on the ward, so you're safe. I can get you a room by yourself if you want.

Randall
They're going to cut mine off, too.

Dr. Hughes
I know. Are you okay with that?

Randall
I don't know.

Dr. Hughes

You'll be under anesthesia, so it won't hurt. But when you wake up you'll have to take pain killers for a while.

Randall

I know. Dr. Jason told me.

Dr. Hughes

But he scared you, didn't he?

Randall

Yes, my mother told him to.

> (*There's a commotion outside the door. We hear Jack yelling.*)

Jack
(*O. S.*)

Where is my son? No, leave me alone. Get off me!! I want to find my son.

Dr. Hughes
(*Sticking her head out the door.*)

Mr. Bender, we're in here.

Jack
(*O.S.*)

Where the hell is that?

> (*He's peeking through the window in the door.*)

My God!! What kind of a room is that?

Dr. Hughes
(*Yelling through the door.*)

I'll be right out to speak with you.

> (*Randall has curled back into a fetal position and he is rocking back and forth.*)

Randall, I'm so sorry. I'll take care of it, I promise.

> **Act 2: Scene 4:** Jack and Meg are at home arguing again.
> **At rise:** They are seated across from each other in the kitchen.

Jack
It's pathetic. Our boy in a padded cell. Curled up in a ball for God's sake.

Meg
He used to curl up like that a lot when he was little.

Jack
He got over that after I taught him chess.

Meg
They go backward and forward. I guess he's going backward.

Jack
You shouldn't have called . . .

Meg
Shut up, Jack! Don't tell me I shouldn't have anything. I was trying to save his life.

Jack
I could've helped him.

Meg
No, you couldn't have! You agreed to it, too. Don't be blaming me. Remember what the doctor said.

Jack
Why do things have to be like this? Couldn't we just have a normal son?

Meg
Cut it out. You know we had to give up "normal" a long time ago.

Jack

I don't want to give up normal! Why should I? My brother has normal kids. They get married, have kids of their own. They don't ask to change their sex or fall in love with trailer park trash.

Meg

Oh, I'm so tired of your complaints. You're so old-fashioned. Don't you watch the news and see what's going on? A lot of people are changing their sex.

Jack

Not autistic people. I don't care what you say. I don't want my son doing this.

Meg

He's already decided. And the doctors are helping him.

Jack

That's why I want to get him out of there.

Meg

Didn't you trust Dr. Hughes? I thought she was great. When she feels it's safe for Randall to come home, she'll send him home.

Jack

Doctors make mistakes too. She's not God, you know. They'll send him home castrated. You want that?

Meg

Dr. Jason told me they can leave most of the penis there and create around it.

Jack

So you're into it now?

Meg

I just want Randall to be happy.

Jack

That's ridiculous! You didn't even want him circumcised and now you're into this?

Meg

I didn't want my baby to suffer that pain. He couldn't make a choice as an infant, but now he's choosing what he wants.

Jack

It went against my upbringing and my religion to leave him uncircumcised, but I did what you wanted, but not this.

Meg

That's the only thing I've done against you, Jack. You know I always try to please you and at the same time I'm trying to help Randall. The two of you are pulling me apart. I'm such an idiot to try and accommodate everyone.

Jack

Let me ask you, Meg, are you just doing what's fashionable?

Meg

Of course not. How absurd!

Jack

Well, you're saying it's what everyone's doing. I don't want to do what everyone else is doing. I remember that time when you worked at St. Mary's and everyone was wearing those stupid wedge flip-flops. You got a pair, and then you fell and broke your leg.

Meg

You remember the worst things! Why don't you remember how well I did there in my first year as a social worker?

Jack

I remember how I had to carry you into the car. I loved that you relied on me like that.

Meg

You liked me to be so helpless.

Jack

Yes, I did! And we got married shortly after that.

Meg

So you're saying you want a helpless woman who relies on you? Maybe that's why Randall wants to be a woman. He feels helpless, and you've encouraged that in me and in him.

Jack

What? I'm not saying that. I'm only saying that we should stick with our individuality and not try to follow some trends or fashions, especially when it concerns destroying our bodies.

Meg

I know. You're an individual. You always have to be different. Where has that gotten us? We don't have many friends. We don't socialize with our neighbors. We're practically outcasts in the neighborhood.

Jack

That's not true! And you? You want to destroy our son to be popular?

Meg

Of course not!! I'm not destroying our son! I'm trying to see things from his point of view.

Jack

Forget it! You could never see things from his point of view. He's got an IQ of 90, even though he's a chess whiz. I don't know how he does that.

Meg

Why are you so against this, Jack? I just don't understand.

Jack

I've thought about that a lot. It's not just a knee-jerk reaction. If I told you what happened to me. . . . Maybe I should tell you . . .

Meg

Tell me what? For the twenty-five years we've been married you've told me so many things. What could you possibly have left out?

Jack

OK, I'll tell you. You know I went to camp as a kid.

Meg

You've told me enough stories about that. I think I even remember your bunkmate's name. Chaim or something like that.

Jack

It was Chaim. And the counselor was David, a handsome Adonis if there ever was one. One night David called me into his cabin. He said he wanted to show me something. I was honored to be chosen by him. We all idealized him. He pulled out these dirty magazines. Then he grabbed me and. . . . That's why I hate *fagelas*! Do you get it? I hate them!! And my son isn't even that. He's going to become something worse, something so weird, so perverted . . .

Meg

Oh, Jack, I'm so sorry to hear that happened to you. You were raped. That's just . . .

Jack

I didn't even run away. I just lay there and took it. I might have even enjoyed it. I hated myself after. I didn't tell anyone. I was so ashamed. I didn't even tell you.

Meg

It wasn't your fault. You were 13 or 14? You should have told someone.

Jack

I blame myself. I think I gave Randall my genes, my fagela genes.

Meg

I don't think it has to do with genes.

Jack

What else is it?

(*The landline phone rings. Meg pounces on it.*)

Meg

Hello? Who? No, he's not! Don't you ever call here again.

> (*Jack grabs the phone out of her hand.*)

Jack

Who is this? Who?!! What do you want? Do you know what harm you've done to our son? Do you know that . . .
She hung up!! That bitch hung up on me!

Meg

What nerve she has to call here.

Jack

That's it! She's got a hold on Randall, and she doesn't want to let go. It's all her fault. I don't think he would have come up with a sex change idea if she hadn't talked him into it.

Meg

Her son turned into a daughter. Randall told me that she recommended the clinic he went to . . .

Jack

I knew he couldn't have come up with that by himself.

Meg

If she comes back here, I'll

Jack

And I'll help you!

> **Act 2, Scene 5**: Randall has had the sex change operation.
> **At rise**: He is lying in bed in the hospital, receiving visitors. Meg is by his side.

Meg
(*Holding Randall's hand.*)
Your breathing sounds funny. Should I call the nurse?

Randall
No, Mom, I'm fine. A little stuffed up is all. I was told I was in surgery for five hours.

Meg
I was terrified something had gone wrong, but they said it's just a delicate operation.

Randall
Thank you for being with me. Where's Dad?

Meg
He went to do something with his car. He should be here soon, I hope.

Randall
Is he OK ...

Meg
He better be.

> (*She fusses around him, adjusting sheets, making sure his monitors are plugged in.*)

Randall
I feel good. A little sore. Not as bad as Dr. Jason said.

Meg
Please forgive me.

Randall
Of course, Mom.

> (*They hold hands and look into each others' eyes.*)

Meg

I just want you to be happy. I was so scared something would go wrong.

Randall

I love you.

Meg
(*Crying.*)

Oh, Randall. My baby.

> (*They hug.*)

Patricia
(*Enters.*)

Well, hello! How's my girlfriend?

> (*Meg jumps up.*)

Meg

You can't be here!

Patricia

I sure feel like I am (*pats herself down*). Yep. One hundred percent here, in the flesh.

Randall
(*Trying to sit up.*)

Patty! You came back! Ouchhh!!

Patricia

I wouldn't miss this for anything.

> (She kisses Randall and plops
> down in the chair opposite Meg.)

Meg

You should have stayed in L.A. where you belong.

Patricia

Mom is watching the kids. I had some extra bucks, so I came.

Meg

After what you did . . .

Patricia

Oh, lay off me, lady. Randall can use all the help he can get now.

Meg

He doesn't need your help, thank you.

Randall

Yes, I do, Mom, I need her help.

Patricia

That's a boy, sorry, a girl! How you feeling, Randy?

Randall

Really fine.

> (*He coughs and can't stop. Meg and Patricia both look upset.*)

Meg

That doesn't sound good at all.

Patricia

Don't fuss so much. You gotta leave kids alone, or you make them nervous.

Meg

Thanks for your parenting advice, but my concern is real.

Patricia

I'm sure it is. Just trying to help.

Meg

I resent you being here at a time like this.

Randall

Mom, you don't understand. I want Patricia here.

Meg

Really, Randall? After all you've been through?

Randall

People who love me—around me—that's the best.

Patricia

The tarot cards said all your stars are aligned perfectly for this operation to be a success.

Meg

What the hell does that mean?

Randall

She reads tarot cards and does astrology.

Meg

That figures!

Patricia

I don't want to tell you what the cards said about you and your husband.

Meg

Thank you.

(Her phone rings. She answers.)

Hi, Jack. You're here?
Excuse me.

(She exits.)

Patricia
(Laughing.)

I'm so glad to see you!

(They kiss.)

Now that big mama is gone we can have some fun. You're gonna be my girl-friend forever! I'll take you back to L.A. with me.

Randall

Would that be OK with your mom?

Patricia

Nothin' is OK with her. I might just stick a tent under the freeway like every-body else I know. I could live there with you and the kids.

Randall

I don't know. What about a shower?

Patricia

Who needs that? We'll just have fun.

Randall

I like to shower.

Patricia

Ah come on. I'm sure that they have some kind of facility for it.

Randall

I'm going to play in the Women's World Chess Championship.

Patricia

That a girl!!! I know you're so good at chess.

Randall

I'm almost at the Expert level.

Patricia

I hope they don't give you any trouble about being a woman; after all, you had the operation.

Randall

It's in Switzerland at the end of the year.

Patricia

They gave transwomen trouble at the Olympics and other sports events. Switzerland is pretty far from L.A., baby.

Randall

I'll leave from here. It's 5,764 miles from Phoenix. It will take 12 hours.

Patricia

You want to go without me?

Randall

I want to go. You can come with me if you want.

Patricia

Hey, wait a minute. Are you saying what I think you are? Remember I sold my RV to come back here and be with you.

Randall

I've been really thinking.

Patricia

Don't think too much. It's bad for your head.
Anyway. What's under these covers?

> (*She lifts the sheet up and peeks.*)

Just like my daughter was, all covered up in bandages.
Does it hurt, honey?

> (*Randall nods and grabs her hand away before she can tickle him.*)

Randall

Don't touch.

Patricia

I won't. Don't worry so much. You're acting strange. Maybe it was the anesthesia.

Randall

As soon as I can move around . . .

Patricia

Wait. I hear them coming back. Watch this.

> (*She slips under the bed and stays there when Jack and Meg reenter.*)

Randall
(*Giggling.*)

What are you . . .?

Jack
(*Enters yelling.*)
Get the hell away from him now!! Where is she?

> (*He looks around for Patricia, but
> doesn't see her anywhere.*)

Meg
(*Enters behind him.*)
I don't know. . . . She was just here a minute ago.

Jack

You said she was here.

Meg

Well, she was, wasn't she, Randall?

Randall

Hello, Mom, Dad, please sit down. Don't fight.

> (*Jack hurries over to the bedside.*)

Jack

How are you, son?

Randall

Remember, Dad . . .

Jack

Oh, yeah. That's going to take some getting used to.

Randall

I'm OK.

Jack

Are you in pain?

Randall

Not so much if I don't move.

Jack

We'll take good care of you at home.

Randall

Thank you.

Jack

Was that woman here, bothering you?

Randall

She doesn't bother me, Dad. She makes me feel good.

Meg

Don't we do that?

Randall

No.

Jack

Oh, Randall, don't say that. We try so hard to . . .

Randall

Dr. Hughes said you mean well, but I have to try and be on my own more.

Jack

First you have to heal up. Being on your own wouldn't be too bad then.

Meg

We only want the best for you.

Randall

I told Patricia that I'm going to play in the Women's World Chess Championship in Switzerland.

Jack

What an idea.

Meg

Maybe we can go with him there, Jack.

Jack

Maybe. We haven't been to Switzerland for a long time.

Meg

First get well and then we'll see.

Randall

I think I'd like to go alone.

Jack

Do you think you can . . .

> (*Patricia pulls on Jack's pants leg from under the bed.*)

What the hell!!! Is that a rat under there?

> (*Jack and Meg both freak out while Randall giggles. Patricia pops up suddenly.*)

Patricia

Surprise!! You were looking for me?

Meg

Not really!! What were you . . .

Jack

There you are!! Get out now!!

Randall

She's only having fun, Dad.

Patricia

That's what you all need! Some good fun.

Meg

How old are you that you were hiding under the bed!? I mean . . .

Patricia

I know how to have fun. And that's just what Randy needs, to have fun, to enjoy his life. You people are so stuffy and stuck up.

Jack

You're judging us?!! Leave before I call . . .

Patricia

Who you gonna call? They'll ask Randy if she wants me here, and she's gonna say yes. Why don't you both leave?

Randall

Please, just stop fighting everyone!

Meg

OK. Let's all leave. It's a good idea to just let Randall have some quiet time by himself, herself, I mean.

> (*She winks at Jack and grabs his arm to walk him out of the room.*)

Jack

Well, no, I mean. . . . Only if Patricia comes with us.

Patricia

Nobody's telling me what to do. I'm staying.

Randall

I would like everyone to leave. Like Mom said.

Patricia

Really, Randy?

Randall

Yes, please.

> (*He pulls out a miniature chess set*
> *and sets up the pieces on the bed.*
> *They all stare at him.*)

THE END

I was interested in how families react to this change of identity. If you know a person as a male or a female, that identity and your behavior toward him or her are usually locked into your mind. The first question most parents ask when a baby is born is: Is it a boy or a girl? Gender determines so many issues in our societies. So, change of gender disrupts set patterns of behavior that we have followed for centuries: for instance, which groups people are allowed into, what educational options, what professions, as well as which socioeconomic status levels, political connections, religious affiliations, and more are considered gender appropriate.

Our societies are changing so rapidly due in part to these changes in identities. Some countries will not permit gender alterations. They rigidly reinforce the male/female dyad. In our present world, strict adherence to male/female differences mostly encourages males to dominate females so that women are given less power, receive less education, are able to accrue fewer goods of high value, and other things. This ancient practice of restricting females from working and from political power produces more children in the world. I believe that we are changing in part because we realize that we have overpopulated our world (either consciously or unconsciously) and need to drastically slow down human reproduction. What better way to do this than to let males become females and females become males? Shakespeare could only write this as a plot twist, but we can perform these transformations in real life. Usually, when people have sex changes, they are not fertile afterward. Of course, transsexuals account for only a small percentage of the population at this time, but the concepts involved with these gender changes are powerful for society and force us to reconsider all our gender prejudices.

Besides gender identity, there is age identity, which is hardly addressed in our present society. But theater, which usually can offset our collective blind spots by confronting important or controversial issues well before they are acknowledged by society as a whole, may function as a very powerful harbinger of change, especially in volatile, vulnerable, or disturbing areas of human awareness.

Certainly, in our present time at least, gender identity issues would fall into the red flag category of "most threatening" to the status quo. Ageism, artificial intelligence, brain transplantation, organ regeneration from stem cells, and other life-span issues hovering on the horizon have only now begun to appear on the planet's human radar screen. What comes next in the world of megamorphing human identity changes—whether from an alien invasion or—remains to be seen. But whatever the case may be in the foreseeable future, perhaps our "Theater of the Absurd" is not so absurd after all!

14

What We Learn From Plays

As I was preparing to write this book, I leafed through hundreds of playbills. Had I really seen so many plays in the last ten years? I thought, what makes a play great? What makes a play even memorable? Is it psychological drama? Is it remarkable characters? Is it pure shock value? Simple plots? Complicated ones? Good actors? The answer was elusive. I know I remembered the plays by Shakespeare that I'd seen. Was it because they were so famous and I'd seen them so many times in so many films, plays, and stories? Or, was it that the Bard had mined the real treasures of the human condition? I remembered the George Bernard Shaw plays as well, and those by Tennessee Williams and Eugene O'Neill.

Jerusalem by Jez Butterworth also stayed with me, even though I'd seen that one in 2011. In the Broadway version, Mark Rylance, a great actor, plays Johnny "Rooster" Byron, a daredevil biker who lives in a trailer and supplies the neighborhood with drugs and alcohol. Of course, the council officials want to evict him, but he holds out. I think he is so memorable because he represents our id, the unconscious primitive part of us that just wants sex, drugs, and rock and roll. Most of the proper people who meet him are the superego characters. A few people are the mediating ego characters. *Jerusalem* is a very important hymn for English people. They sing it in sports stadiums, churches, and other gathering places. William Blake, one of their finest poets, wrote it in 1804. It supposes that Jesus traveled to England, a heaven on Earth. Blake wrote that they wouldn't stop fighting until a Jerusalem was built in England. The poem became a song that helped British soldiers fight in World War I. Johnny "Rooster" in the play crows this song, offering optimism and life to what the playwright sees as a dying England.

Many playwrights enjoy retelling the plays of the masters, like the Greeks and Shakespeare. One could bring to mind, for instance, *Rosencrantz and Guildenstern Are Dead* by Tom Stoppard and *Fool* by Christopher Moore, to name just two pieces that are trying to retell Shakespeare. Why do they do it? Perhaps if it's a conscious effort, it assures the playwright that his or her work will be considered of a higher order and taken seriously.

I believe Tom Stoppard in *Rosencrantz and Guildenstern Are Dead* (1964) is consciously aware that he is taking two minor characters from *Hamlet* and giving them major roles. In *Hamlet*, these two characters are under the king's command and sidelined to spy on Hamlet, but Hamlet outwits both of them and maneuvers them to their deaths. Rosencrantz and Guildenstern have no idea what's going on in Stoppard's play. They are unconscious of Hamlet's deeds because he's a minor character to them. People were entranced with this play and saw the absurdity as an exercise in probability theory, as a metaphor for art versus reality. They projected all kinds of meaning on Stoppard's play.

Fool (2009) by Christopher Moore is a modern retelling of *King Lear*. It's a novel about the madness of Lear and Pocket, his fool, who sets out to clean up Lear's mess. Moore says he borrowed from many of Shakespeare's plays in his writing. It has become a play.

Mimicry is an essential part of human behavior. All primates copy each other's behavior, and we are no exception. Copying others has social benefits: Groups bond, and individuals have rapport with each other, but in literature, if it goes too far, it's called plagiarism. Neither Stoppard nor Moore plagiarized Shakespeare. They just took his characters and developed them in their own way.

Mirroring is the unconscious imitation of another person. We do this when speaking and with certain behaviors. Mirror neurons in our brain are activated when we hear another person talking or see them behaving in a certain way. This enables us to have a greater understanding of other people. Why does Tom Stoppard mirror Shakespeare? It could be because English was not the language he was born into. He was born in Czechoslovakia, and the family left when he was a child to escape the Nazis. His family went to India and then Britain. English was his second language, and he probably admired the Bard, who was so agile and clever in his new language. Stoppard also wanted to play with the English language. What better way was there than to take Shakespeare's characters and use them as he would?

Clybourne Park (2010) by Bruce Norris addresses issues that started with Lorraine Hansberry's play *A Raisin in the Sun* (1959). *Clybourne* starts act 1 in 1959, when a grieving white couple wants to sell their house in a white middle-class neighborhood to a Black family. Their clergyman, Jim, and neighbors beg them not to. The family moving in will be the Youngers, from *A Raisin*. The white couple don't care that their neighbors are against this because the neighbors didn't care that their son had committed suicide after returning from the Korean War. Act 2 is set in 2009 in the same house, but the same actors play different characters. Clybourne Park is now a Black neighborhood that is gentrifying. A white couple wants to buy the house, and they plan major renovations. The Black housing board is unwilling to allow this, and there is an argument about racial issues. Steve, of the white couple, feels they are being discriminated against. They find the suicide note of the son who died back in 1957.

All in all, this play is about the changing values/mores of society and about discrimination from each group, but the play is also another one spinning off from an established work—namely, Hansberry's *Raisin*. In the case of *Clybourne Park*, I can understand why the playwright gives us the two time periods to show us that in 50 years not much has changed. We are still fighting discrimination battles, even when situations reverse.

In *As You Like It*, act 1 (1599), by William Shakespeare, Orlando, the youngest son of the recently deceased Sir Roland de Boys, is treated badly by his eldest brother, Oliver. An angry Orlando challenges the court wrestler, Charles, to a fight. His brother, Oliver, tells Charles to injure Orlando as much as he can. Duke Frederick has recently deposed his brother, Duke Senior, as head of the court. Senior's daughter, Rosalind, remains behind. When Rosalind and Celia (the new duke's daughter and Rosalind's cousin) watch the wrestling match, Rosalind falls in love with Orlando, who beats Charles. Rosalind gives Orlando a chain to wear, and he falls in love with her.

In act 2, Orlando is warned of his brother's plot against him and seeks refuge in the Forest of Arden. At the same time, and seemingly without cause, Duke Frederick banishes Rosalind. Rosalind flees her uncle's court with Celia to the Forest of Arden. Rosalind disguises herself as the young man Ganymede and Celia as his shepherdess sister, Aliena. Touchstone, the court fool, also goes with them.

In act 3, in the Forest of Arden the weary cousins meet Silvius, a lovesick shepherd. Silvius was telling Phoebe about his love, but she scorns him. Ganymede buys the lease to the property of an old shepherd who needs someone to manage his estate. Ganymede and Aliena set up home in the forest. Not far away, and unaware of them, Duke Senior is living a simple outdoor life with his fellow outlawed men. Orlando arrives, needing food for himself and his servant. They are welcomed by the outlaw courtiers.

Ganymede and Aliena find verses addressed to Rosalind hung on the forest branches by Orlando. Ganymede runs into Orlando and wants to cure him of his love. Ganymede proposes that Orlando will woo him or her as if he were Rosalind (even though "he" really is Rosalind). Orlando consents and visits Ganymede/Rosalind every day for his lessons. In the meantime, the shepherdess Phoebe has fallen for Ganymede, while the shepherd, Silvius, still loves her. Furthermore, Touchstone, the court fool, has dazzled a country girl, Audrey, with his courtly manners. Audrey deserts her young suitor, William, for him.

Act 4 has Duke Frederick learning that Orlando disappeared at the same time as Rosalind and Celia. Brother Oliver is sent to the forest to seek Orlando. In the forest, Orlando saves Oliver's life, injuring his arm in the process. Oliver runs into Ganymede and Aliena in the forest and tells them this news. Rosalind (still disguised as Ganymede) feels her love for Orlando. Celia (disguised as Aliena) and Oliver quickly fall in love with one another. Rosalind decides that it is time to end her game with Orlando and devises a plan in which everyone will get married.

In act 5, as Ganymede, Rosalind promises Phoebe that they will marry, Celia will marry Oliver, Touchstone will marry Audrey, and Orlando will marry Rosalind. She makes Phoebe promise that if they, for some reason, don't get married, Phoebe will marry Silvius instead.

On the day of the wedding, and with the help of the god Hymen, Rosalind reappears in her female clothes. Duke Senior gives her away to Orlando, while Phoebe accepts Silvius. Orlando's other older brother returns from college with the news that Celia's father, Duke Ferdinand, has left court to become a hermit. Thus, everyone is happy (except maybe Phoebe, who marries someone she doesn't love, and Silvius, who marries someone who doesn't love him). The play ends with a joyful dance to celebrate the four marriages.

Love is the central theme of *As You Like It*, like other romantic comedies of Shakespeare. Following the tradition of a romantic comedy, it is a tale of love manifested in its varied forms. In many of the love couples, it is "love at first sight" (e.g., Rosalind and Orlando, Celia and Oliver, as well as Phebe and Ganymede). The love story of Audrey and Touchstone is a parody of romantic love. Another form of love is between women, as in Rosalind and Celia's deep bond.

Gender is another one of the play's important themes. While disguised as Ganymede, Rosalind disrupts the social norms of her times. Rosalind is demanding and disobedient. By claiming that women who are wild are smarter than those who are not, Rosalind refutes the perception of women as passive in their pursuit of men.

In this play, it is Jaques, a melancholy clown, who explains life. He is able to "break the fourth wall" and interpret what is happening on stage. He drones on about the sadness of life and sees the world through black-tinted lenses. This perspective allows him to understand the various stages of life, as described in the famous passage: "All the world's a stage." This particular Shakespearean character, while not bipolar, is definitely depressed.

When I reveal that I am not only a psychiatrist but also a writer and artist, many people become skeptical and annoyed. The attitude seems to be that I have strayed beyond my boundaries, and I should pick one of these and be done with it. It's understandable because there is so much information, people wonder how I can be proficient in three areas. What they fail to realize is that a person can never have all the information anyway—whether they defined themselves as a writer, painter, or even a psychiatrist or, God forbid, all three! I don't want to be squeezed into one box and prefer the interdisciplinary approach.

During the Renaissance, creators such as Leonardo da Vinci took on many roles. He was an artist, engineer, architect, and scientist as well as an inventor. The Renaissance spanned the period from the fourteenth through the seventeenth century. It was the transition from the Middle Ages to the modern age. There was a blossoming of interest in science, art, and literature. Da Vinci was a polymath, and no one questioned him about it. In modern times, we have such polymath titans as Oliver Sachs, Anton Chekhov, and Albert Einstein. Their contributions have, in fact, opened up new areas of inquiry and enhanced the various fields in which each of these modern-day, multifaceted geniuses excelled.

We may believe that breaking the fourth wall in theater is new, but it's not. The convention assumes that there is an invisible wall between the audience and the actors. The audience sees through the wall to the performance, but presumably the actors can't see the audience. The famous Russian director Konstantin Stanislavski (1863–1938) believed in the fourth wall and called it "public solitude." He wanted his actors to totally get into their roles and believe and feel the reality of the play. Down through the centuries from classical Greek theater to the plays of the European Renaissance, actors frequently addressed the audience with asides and monologues.

Breaking the fourth wall is when actors address the audience directly. *Fleabag* consists of one long soliloquy, and so does *Hamlet* (Chapter 2). We get to hear the characters' most intimate thoughts and feelings. In *Fleabag*, there are no other characters except the main one, so we travel with her through her many adventures. In *Hamlet*, there are many other characters, but Shakespeare wanted us to understand what was really happening in

Hamlet's mind. Shakespeare frequently had his actors address the audience, providing comic relief. He also used the device of "plays within plays" in several pieces (i.e., *A Midsummer Night's Dream*).

In modern theater, playwrights wanted realism, so they broke the fourth wall. We see this in Wilder's *Our Town* and in plays by Ibsen, Strindberg, and Chekhov.

There is always "the suspension of disbelief" when we are viewing a play. We have to believe what the playwright is showing us. If we are thrown out of our suspension of disbelief, we don't enjoy the play. Our minds wander away from the story. When a character breaks the fourth wall and addresses us directly, we usually have one of two reactions. One, we can dive more deeply into the story because we delve into that person's mind. Or two, we can disengage from the story being told. In a way, the playwright forces us to see the duality of watching his or her play by taking us out of the play's original worldview. However, with our suspension of disbelief, we are still able to remain immersed in the playwright's tale.

Theater is having a revival in New York City now that the pandemic is almost becoming endemic. I was worried that we would just Zoom all our shows. Live theater improves empathy, changes attitudes, and shapes many of our behaviors, not to mention that it creates new neural networks in our brains. May theater live on for many eons.

Chart of Plays that Won Tonys

Item No.	Playbill Date	Theater	Name of Play	Playwright(s)	Psychiatric Condition
1	2015 January	Lyceum NYC	DISGRACED	Ayad Akhtar	Systemic racism, ethnic prejudice, paranoia (PD)
2	2014 November	Ethel Barrymore NYC	THE CURIOUS INCIDENT OF THE DOG IN THE NIGHT-TIME	Simon Stephens	Autism
3	2012 August	The Duke on 42nd Street NYC	COCK	Mike Bartlett	Male aggression and competition
4	2006 February	The Duke on 42nd Street, NYC	ALL'S WELL THAT ENDS WELL	William Shakespeare	
5	2005 June	Booth theatre, NYC	THE PILLOWMAN	Martin McDonagh	Sociopathy Sadistic Personality Disorder
6*	2003	Neighborhood Playhouse NYC	UNDER THE DRAGON	Carol W. Berman	Schizoaffective Disorder
7	2017 May	John Golden Theater NYC	THE DOLL'S HOUSE PART 2	Lucas Hnath	Personality Disorder
8	2017 May	Court Theater NYC	INDECENT	Paula Vogel	Lesbianism
9	2011 July	Music Box NYC	JERUSALEM	Jez Butterworth	Sociopathy
10	2009 April	St. James NYC	DESIRE UNDER THE ELMS	Eugene O' Neill	Oedipus Complex
11	2010 February	Atlantic Theater Company	AGNES OF THE MOON	Sam Shepard	Male aggression & Competion
12	2009 July	Booth NYC	NEXT TO NORMAL	Tom Kitt and Yorkey	Bipolar Disorder
13	2011	Riverside Theater	ORESTEIA	Aeschylus	Electra Complex

* play written by author of this book

Chart of Plays that Show Psychiatric Conditions

Item No.	Playbill Date	Theater	Name of Play	Playwright(s)	Psychiatric Condition
1	2015 January	Lyceum NYC	DISGRACED	Ayad Akhtar with Danny Ashok and Karen Pittman	Systemic racism, ethnic prejudice, paranoia (PD)
2	2014 November	Ethel Barrymore NYC	THE CURIOUS INCIDENT OF THE DOG IN THE NIGHT-TIME	Simon Stephens	Autism
3	2012 August	The Duke on 42nd Street NYC	COCK	Mike Bartlett	
4	2006 February	The Duke on 42nd Street NYC	ALL'S WELL THAT ENDS WELL	William Shakespeare	
5	2005 June		THE PILLOWMAN	Martin McDonagh	Sociopathy Sadistic Personality Disorder
6*	2003		UNDER THE DRAGON	Carol W. Berman	Schizoaffective Disorder
7	2017 May	John Golden Theater NYC	THE DOLL'S HOUSE PART 2	Lucas Hnath	Personality Disorder
8	2017 May	Court Theater NYC	INDECENT	Paula Vogel	Lesbianism
9	2011 July	Music Box NYC	JERUSALEM	Jez Butterworth	Sociopathy
10	2009 April	St. James NYC	DESIRE UNDER THE ELMS	Eugen O'Neill	Oedipus Complex
11	2010 February	Atlantic Theater Company	AGNES OF THE MOON	Sam Shepard	
12	2009 July	Booth NYC	NEXT TO NORMAL	Tom Kitt and Yorkey	Bipolar Disorder
13	2009 April		ORESTEIA	Aeskhulos Sophocles Euripides	Electra Complex

* play written by author of this book

Index